Last Minute
Meals for
People with Diabetes

Nancy S. Hughes

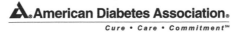

American Diabetes Association®
Cure • Care • Commitment™

Director, Book Publishing, John Fedor; *Associate Director, Consumer Books,* Sherrye L. Landrum; *Editor,* Laurie Guffey; *Production Manager,* Peggy M. Rote; *Composition,* Circle Graphics, Inc.; *Cover Design,* VC Graphics, Inc.; *Printer,* Port City Press.

Printed in the United States of America
1 3 5 7 9 10 8 6 4 2

The suggestions and information contained in this publication are generally consistent with the *Clinical Practice Recommendations* and other policies of the American Diabetes Association, but they do not represent the policy or position of the Association or any of its boards or committees. Reasonable steps have been taken to ensure the accuracy of the information presented. However, the American Diabetes Association cannot ensure the safety or efficacy of any product or service described in this publication. Individuals are advised to consult a physician or other appropriate health care professional before undertaking any diet or exercise program or taking any medication referred to in this publication. Professionals must use and apply their own professional judgment, experience, and training and should not rely solely on the information contained in this publication before prescribing any diet, exercise, or medication. The American Diabetes Association—its officers, directors, employees, volunteers, and members—assumes no responsibility or liability for personal or other injury, loss, or damage that may result from the suggestions or information in this publication.

♾ The paper in this publication meets the requirements of the ANSI Standard Z39.48-1992 (permanence of paper).

ADA titles may be purchased for business or promotional use or for special sales. For information, please write to Lee Romano Sequeira, Special Sales & Promotions, at the address below.

American Diabetes Association
1701 North Beauregard Street
Alexandria, Virginia 22311

Library of Congress Cataloging-in-Publication Data
Hughes, Nancy S., 1950–
    Last minute meals / Nancy S. Hughes.
        p. cm.
    Includes index.
    ISBN 1-58040-082-5 (pbk. : alk. paper)
    1. Diabetes—Diet therapy—Recipes. 2. Quick and easy cookery. I. Title.
    RC662 .H84 2002
    641.5'6314—dc21

                                                                                                     2002018322

Dedication

To my husband, Greg,
my best friend, the other side of my brain.

To my son, Will, 25,
whose culinary passion took off,
and who now shares the passion of the trade.

To my daughter, Annie, 22,
whose caring heart helped me see the reader behind the recipes.

To my son, Taft, 17,
who finds the calm for me when things get wild around the house.

I quietly thank you.

Contents

Preface

"**I just want to GET IN and GET OUT of that kitchen!**" How many times have you felt like that? This book was created for people like you who want to stay on the go, but also eat healthfully. Whether you are diagnosed with diabetes, cooking for someone who has diabetes, or just want to eat better by taking control of your carbohydrates, this book is exactly what you need.

You might feel that changing to healthier eating habits is overwhelming, aggravating, and, basically, too much trouble. You don't want, nor do you have the time, to shop for specialty foods, hunt down special sections in the grocery store, or buy a lot of strange ingredients. You want your meat AND your potatoes AND your cake, too. You want normal food, just like everyone else. You don't want to walk around with a calculator, a carb-counting book, or perform a juggling act in your head every time you want to eat. And you don't want to starve to death while you're waiting for dinner to be ready!

If you feel like this, you're holding the right cookbook! My goal was to develop recipes that would not tax the brain or require a lot of energy to prepare, but still provide great-tasting, home-cooked meals. A home-cooked meal, after all, does soothe the mind, body and soul . . . but NOT if it takes up your last drop of energy. I intentionally created and tested every recipe when I was tired . . . yes, really tired. At the end of each day, with pan in hand, I took a deep breath and started in. Not only are these recipes simple and fast, but they are economical and easy to clean up. Best of all, they have six ingredients or less (not counting seasonings) . . . that means they ARE really simple, really fast, really economical, and really easy to clean up.

You CAN have normal food and still be in control of your diabetes and your health. Every recipe has nutritional info such as carb, calorie, and sodium counts listed so you can stay within your personal guidelines. (Remember that the nutritional analysis does not include optional ingredients.) Since these meals are for everyone, you'll be eating the same food as your family and friends. You'll like this, not only because there's less hassle in making one meal instead of two, but because you don't have to feel singled out because of diabetes.

With a **maximum** of six ingredients and a **minimum** amount of effort, you can get in and out of that kitchen and get on with your life (and have more fun while you're at it!).

Enjoy!

Acknowledgments

Thanks to my editors at ADA, Laurie Guffey and Sherrye Landrum, who stopped their busy worlds for me whenever I called, listened with enthusiasm, and believed in me and encouraged others to do the same.

And thanks to Sarees Zieman, whose dependability and positive attitude made our work a joy from initial recipe concepts through final testings. You were always there smiling for me.

Stress-Free Starters and Snacks

This chapter contains recipes that are easy for any occasion, from watching a Friday night video to entertaining by candlelight. Many of these recipes may be made in advance and refrigerated to have on hand whenever you get the urge! Keep in mind that you can use fresh veggies and fruits with any dip recipe that suggests chips or bread.

Be creative with the varieties of vegetables and fruits you use, too. For instance, use yellow squash or cucumbers cut diagonally instead of in sliced rounds, or blanch whole green beans or asparagus spears for dipping. Or hollow out the center of an acorn squash and fill it to the brim with dip for your next party. It's an easy way to dress up your table.

These recipes can go away from home, too! Try taking them to work or tossing them in a lunch bag for a nice change. And healthy snacks sure come in handy when you see those fast food billboards flashing by on long car trips. Just pack them in disposable plastic containers and you're on your way.

Pizza Mushrooms

This is a safe way to satisfy those pizza cravings!

PREPARATION TIME
12 minutes

SERVES
4

SERVING SIZE
4 mushrooms

16 large whole mushrooms, stems removed
 3 Tbsp bottled pizza sauce
1/4 cup grated reduced-fat Mozzarella cheese (1 oz)

1. Heat oven to 475°F.
2. Arrange mushrooms on a nonstick baking sheet and spray mushrooms with cooking spray. Spoon about 1/2 tsp of the pizza sauce in the center of each mushroom. Sprinkle mozzarella evenly over mushrooms, about a scant tsp per mushroom.
3. Bake 5 minutes or until mushrooms are tender and cheese is lightly golden. Remove from oven and let stand 5 minutes to absorb flavors and cool slightly.

Exchanges

1 Vegetable

1/2 Fat

Calories 45
  Calories from Fat . 15
Total Fat. . . . . 2 g
  Saturated Fat. . . . . . . 1 g
Cholesterol . . . . 4 mg
Sodium . . . . 121 mg
Total Carbohydrate . . 5 g
  Dietary Fiber . . . . 1 g
  Sugars. . . . . 2 g
Protein . . . . 4 g

Roasted Pepper Crostini

The secret to the great flavor in this appetizer is rubbing the toasted, cooled bread slices with raw garlic. This can be made up to 3 days in advance. Store cooled bread slices in an airtight container at room temperature. Place pepper mixture in an airtight container and refrigerate until needed.

PREPARATION TIME
6 minutes

SERVES
4

SERVING SIZE
2 crostini

Exchanges

1/2 Starch

1/2 Fat

Calories 65

   Calories from Fat. . . 23

Total Fat. . . . . 3 g

   Saturated Fat. . . . . . . 1 g

Cholesterol . . . . 0 mg

Sodium . . . . 376 mg

Total Carbohydrate . . 8 g

   Dietary Fiber . . . . 0 g

   Sugars . . . . 1 g

Protein . . . . 2 g

2 oz French bread, preferably baguette-style, cut in 1/4-inch slices (or use regular size French bread, cut into 1/2-inch slices, then cut in half slightly on the diagonal to total 8 pieces)

1/3 cup roasted red peppers, chopped

12 small stuffed Spanish olives, coarsely chopped

1/2 tsp dried basil

1 tsp extra virgin olive oil

1 clove garlic, cut in half crosswise

1. Heat oven to 350°F.
2. Place bread slices on nonstick baking sheet and lightly coat bread with cooking spray. Bake 10–12 minutes or until slightly golden around edges. Remove from oven and allow to cool completely.
3. Meanwhile, toss peppers with olives, basil, and oil and set aside.
4. Rub garlic over each slice of cooled bread and top with 1 Tbsp of the pepper mixture.

Pepperoni Pinwheels

Serve these pinwheels at room temperature for the best flavor. Store leftovers in an airtight container.

PREPARATION TIME
15 minutes

SERVES
10

SERVING SIZE
2 pinwheels

Exchanges

1 Starch

1/2 Fat

Calories	107
Calories from Fat . . .	26
Total Fat	3 g
Saturated Fat	1 g
Cholesterol	7 mg
Sodium	299 mg
Total Carbohydrate .	16 g
Dietary Fiber	0 g
Sugars	1 g
Protein	5 g

11 oz pkg French bread dough
1 Tbsp extra virgin olive oil
1 Tbsp dried basil
28 turkey pepperoni slices, coarsely chopped (about 2 oz)
3 oz finely chopped red onion
1/4 cup finely chopped fresh parsley

1. Heat oven to 350°F.
2. Unroll dough on a nonstick baking sheet to form an 11-inch by 15-inch rectangle. Drizzle oil evenly over the dough and spread evenly with your fingertips. Sprinkle with basil, pepperoni, onion, and parsley.
3. Gently roll dough to form a 15-inch log and bake 22–25 minutes or until golden brown.
4. Place on cooling rack and cool completely before slicing. Use a serrated knife and cut into 1/2-inch pieces to serve.

Stuffed Spinach Rolls

Be careful with alfalfa sprouts. They need to be very fresh, purchased from a reliable source, and washed and dried thoroughly before you use them. They can be a source of bacterial infections, so anyone with a weakened immune system should avoid them completely.

PREPARATION TIME
30 minutes

SERVES
4

SERVING SIZE
4 rolls

Exchanges

1 Lean Meat

1 Vegetable

Calories 72
  Calories from Fat . 23
Total Fat . . . . 3 g
  Saturated Fat . . . . . . 1 g
Cholesterol . . . . 12 mg
Sodium . . . . 248 mg
Total Carbohydrate . . 4 g
  Dietary Fiber . . . . . . 2 g
  Sugars . . . . 2 g
Protein . . . . 10 g

16 large spinach leaves, rinsed and pat dry
2 slices reduced-fat Swiss cheese, cut into 16 strips
2 oz oven-roasted deli turkey, cut into 16 strips
1 Tbsp plus 1 tsp honey mustard
1 medium red bell pepper, thinly sliced into 48 strips
1/2 cup alfalfa sprouts
16 wooden toothpicks

1. Place one spinach leaf, smooth side down, on work surface and top with 1 strip of cheese and 1 of turkey. Spread 1/4 tsp mustard evenly over turkey. Top with 3 pepper strips, overlapping slightly, and then 1 1/2 tsp sprouts.
2. Bring sides of spinach to the center, overlapping slightly, forming a roll. Secure diagonally with a wooden toothpick and repeat.

Note: Be sure to line up the ingredients parallel to the center vein of the spinach. Otherwise, it will be difficult to roll and will not resemble a bundle of veggies.

Hot Cheesy Chips

These layered nachos will be a big hit at your next get-together!

PREPARATION TIME
10 minutes

SERVES
8

SERVING SIZE
2 chips

16 baked tortilla chips
1/2 cup grated reduced-fat sharp
      Cheddar cheese (2 oz)
1/2 cup finely chopped poblano chili
      pepper or green bell pepper
1/3 cup chopped ripe olives
1/3 cup reduced-fat sour cream
1/3 cup chopped fresh cilantro

1. Heat oven to 400°F.
2. Place chips on baking sheet and top with equal amounts of cheese, peppers, and olives.
3. Bake 4 minutes or until cheese is melted. Top each with 1 tsp sour cream and 1 tsp cilantro. Serve immediately.

Exchanges

1/2 Carbohydrate

1/2 Fat

Calories 67
  Calories from Fat . 37
Total Fat. . . . . 4 g
  Saturated Fat. . . . . . 2 g
Cholesterol . . . . 8 mg
Sodium . . . . 160 mg
Total Carbohydrate . . 5 g
  Dietary Fiber . . . . 1 g
  Sugars. . . . . 1 g
Protein . . . . 3 g

Triple-Herbed Tomatoes

If you like a more lemony flavor, add an extra 1 Tbsp lemon juice.

PREPARATION TIME
4 minutes

SERVES
7

SERVING SIZE
4 tomatoes

1 pint cherry tomatoes (28), rinsed and patted dry
1 Tbsp lemon juice
1 Tbsp extra virgin olive oil
1 1/2 tsp dried basil
1 tsp dried oregano
1/2 tsp dried tarragon
1/4 tsp salt
1/4 tsp black pepper

Combine all ingredients in a medium bowl and toss until well blended and thoroughly coated.

Exchanges

1 Vegetable

1/2 Fat

Calories 34
  Calories from Fat . 18
Total Fat . . . . 2 g
  Saturated Fat . . . . 0 g
Cholesterol . . . . 0 mg
Sodium . . . . 340 mg
Total Carbohydrate . . 4 g
  Dietary Fiber . . . . 1 g
  Sugars . . . . 2 g
Protein . . . . 1 g

Hummus Dip

For a dramatic look, try dark pumpernickel bread wedges (flatten the bread pieces, cut into triangles, and bake at 350°F for 10 minutes) or pita bread (baked the same way) with this dip.

PREPARATION TIME
5 minutes

SERVES
36

SERVING SIZE
1 piece

1	15-oz can garbanzo beans, rinsed and drained
2/3	cup plain fat-free yogurt
2	cloves garlic, minced
2	Tbsp lime juice
1/2	tsp ground cumin
1/4	tsp salt
36	pieces Melba toast

Combine all ingredients except Melba toast in a blender and blend until smooth. Top each toast piece with 2 tsp dip.

Exchanges

1/2 Starch

Calories 35
  Calories from Fat . . 3
Total Fat. . . . . 0 g
  Saturated Fat. . . . . . . 0 g
Cholesterol . . . . 0 mg
Sodium . . . . 73 mg
Total Carbohydrate . . 6 g
  Dietary Fiber . . . . . . 1 g
  Sugars. . . . . 1 g
Protein . . . . 2 g

Peanutty Dip

Kids love this dip, too!

PREPARATION TIME
5 minutes

SERVES
4

SERVING SIZE
2 Tbsp

3 Tbsp creamy peanut butter
3 Tbsp apricot or orange 100% fruit spread
1 1/2 Tbsp lite soy sauce
2 Tbsp fat-free milk
1/4 tsp ground ginger
24 baby carrots or 2-inch celery sticks or 1/2-inch thick apple slices

In a small mixing bowl, combine all ingredients, except carrots, celery, or apples. Stir until completely blended.

Exchanges

1 Carbohydrate

1 Fat

Calories 121
  Calories from Fat . 56
Total Fat. . . . . 6 g
  Saturated Fat. . . . . . . 1 g
Cholesterol . . . . 0 mg
Sodium . . . . 303 mg
Total Carbohydrate . 14 g
  Dietary Fiber . . . . 2 g
  Sugars . . . . 10 g
Protein . . . . 4 g

Creamy Mustard Dipping Sauce

Serve this dip with broccoli, baby carrots, blanched asparagus, blanched green beans, cauliflower, squash, or cucumbers.

PREPARATION TIME
5 minutes

SERVES
10

SERVING SIZE
1 Tbsp

1/2 cup fat-free buttermilk
3 Tbsp light mayonnaise
1 Tbsp coarse ground mustard or Dijon mustard
1/4 tsp salt
1/8 tsp black pepper

Place all ingredients in a small mixing bowl and whisk together until smooth. Cover with plastic wrap and refrigerate until needed.

Exchanges

1/2 Fat

Calories 21
   Calories from Fat . 15
Total Fat . . . . 2 g
   Saturated Fat . . . . 0 g
Cholesterol . . . . 2 mg
Sodium . . . . 143 mg
Total Carbohydrate . . 1 g
   Dietary Fiber . . . . 0 g
   Sugars . . . . 1 g
Protein . . . . 1 g

Mexicali Dip with Chips

If this dip thickens during serving, return it to the microwave for 30 more seconds.

PREPARATION TIME
5 minutes

SERVES
13

SERVING SIZE
**6 large chips plus
2 Tbsp dip**

8 slices reduced-fat American cheese
1 cup diced fresh tomatoes, patted dry
1 4.5-oz can chopped green chilis
1/2 cup finely chopped green onions
    Hot pepper sauce, to taste
78 baked tortilla chips

1. Place cheese in a medium microwaveable bowl. Cover with plastic wrap and microwave on HIGH setting 60 seconds. Stir and microwave for 30 more seconds.
2. Add tomatoes, chilis, and onions. Stir, cover with wrap, and cook 60 seconds longer or until heated through. Stir in hot sauce, if desired. Serve with tortilla chips.

Exchanges

1/2 Starch

1/2 Fat

Calories 71
  Calories from Fat. . . 20
Total Fat. . . . . 2 g
  Saturated Fat. . . . . . . 1 g
Cholesterol . . . . 6 mg
Sodium . . . . 269 mg
Total Carbohydrate . 10 g
  Dietary Fiber . . . . 2 g
  Sugars . . . . 1 g
Protein . . . . 3 g

Melon with Creamy Dipping Sauce

If you buy precut fruit at the supermarket, use it within 24 hours.

PREPARATION TIME
5 minutes

SERVES
4

SERVING SIZE
1/4 recipe

1/2 cup light sour cream
3 Tbsp powdered sugar
1/2 tsp vanilla
1/4 tsp coconut extract (optional)
1 tsp lime juice
2 cups diced honeydew or cantaloupe melon or seedless grapes or strawberries

1. Combine all ingredients except fruit in a small serving bowl.
2. Place bowl in center of serving platter and arrange fruit around bowl to serve.

Exchanges

1 Fruit

1/2 Fat

Calories 90
 Calories from Fat . . . 25
Total Fat . . . . 3 g
 Saturated Fat . . . . 1 g
Cholesterol . . . . 10 mg
Sodium . . . . 25 mg
Total Carbohydrate . 16 g
 Dietary Fiber . . . . 1 g
 Sugars . . . . 13 g
Protein . . . . 3 g

Sparkling Fruit Smoothies

Try freezing this recipe in ice-cream goblets and serving it as dessert.

PREPARATION TIME
5 minutes

SERVES
4

SERVING SIZE
1/4 recipe

3 cups cold chopped melon or strawberries
1 medium banana
1/2 cup frozen orange-pineapple concentrate
1 12-oz can sugar-free ginger ale

Blend all ingredients until smooth.

Exchanges

2 1/2   Fruit

Calories 159
  Calories from Fat. . . . 1
Total Fat. . . . . 0 g
  Saturated Fat. . . . . . . 0 g
Cholesterol . . . . 0 mg
Sodium . . . . 27 mg
Total Carbohydrate . 37 g
  Dietary Fiber . . . . 4 g
  Sugars . . . . 28 g
Protein . . . . 2 g

Minted Espresso Hot Chocolate

You can make this hot chocolate without coffee if you prefer.

PREPARATION TIME
3 minutes

SERVES
4

SERVING SIZE
1/4 recipe

3 cups fat-free milk
6 Tbsp chocolate syrup
1 Tbsp plus 1 tsp instant coffee granules
1/2 tsp peppermint extract
1/4 cup fat-free whipped topping

1. Place milk, chocolate, and coffee in a medium microwaveable bowl. Cover with plastic wrap and microwave on HIGH for 2 minutes.
2. Stir contents so coffee dissolves and microwave on HIGH for 2 more minutes.
3. Remove from microwave, stir in extract, and pour into 4 individual cups. Top each with 1 Tbsp whipped topping.

Exchanges

2 Carbohydrate

Calories 147
   Calories from Fat 3
Total Fat . . . . 0 g
   Saturated Fat . . . . 0 g
Cholesterol . . . . 3 mg
Sodium . . . . 116 mg
Total Carbohydrate . 29 g
   Dietary Fiber . . . . 0 g
   Sugars . . . . 24 g
Protein . . . . 7 g

No-Chop Salads

The biggest problem with salads is the chopping . . . but you can just leave that knife in the drawer with these recipes. No chopping involved here: just rinse the ingredients, pat dry, and rip apart!

Salads seem to make a meal complete, but it can get rather monotonous if you keep preparing the same salad night after night. Keep variety in mind when you're planning your salads. Color and texture are important factors. Try adding peeled zucchini strips or crunchy red cabbage to your salads. Something as simple as changing from yellow onions to red onions or green peppers to yellow peppers can brighten up a salad.

If you want to give your salad more body, add pre-sliced mushrooms, frozen and thawed green peas, garbanzo beans, or broccoli flowerets. And don't underestimate the power of fresh herbs, such as basil, cilantro, and even parsley. Herbs add zing and enhance the existing flavor of any salad.

It is a great idea to keep several types of salad dressing on hand too. Try drizzling a different dressing than you usually use over sliced cucumbers and tomatoes. Or use them instead of mayonnaise on sandwiches or burgers.

One final tip: opt for the salad when it's your turn to bring a dish, especially if you're like me . . . always running behind schedule!

Torn Crouton Caesar Salad

These croutons may be made 48 hours in advance, cooled, and stored in an airtight container at room temperature.

PREPARATION TIME
5 minutes

SERVES
4

SERVING SIZE
1/4 recipe

Exchanges

1 Carbohydrate

1/2 Fat

Calories 90
   Calories from Fat. . . 33
Total Fat. . . . . 4 g
   Saturated Fat. . . . . . . 1 g
Cholesterol . . . . 6 mg
Sodium . . . . 378 mg
Total Carbohydrate . 11 g
   Dietary Fiber . . . . 1 g
   Sugars . . . . 3 g
Protein . . . . 4 g

1/2 cup fat-free buttermilk
2 Tbsp light mayonnaise
1/8 tsp garlic powder
1/4 tsp salt
1/4 tsp black pepper
2 oz French bread or whole wheat bread, torn gently into 1/2-inch pieces
4 cups pre-packaged mixed greens
1 1/2 Tbsp grated Parmesan cheese

1. Heat oven to 350°F.
2. In a small mixing bowl, whisk together the buttermilk, mayonnaise, garlic powder, salt, and pepper. Cover with plastic wrap and refrigerate at least one hour to thicken slightly.
3. Meanwhile, place bread pieces on baking sheet and bake 12 minutes or until lightly golden. Remove from heat and cool completely.
4. Place mixed greens in a salad bowl, add dressing and cheese, and toss gently, yet thoroughly. Add croutons, toss, and serve.

Romaine and Creamy Dill Dressing

Try this dressing as a dip for fresh vegetables or tossed with cucumber slices for a quick salad.

PREPARATION TIME
3 minutes

SERVES
4

SERVING SIZE
1/4 recipe

1   0.4 oz packet buttermilk salad dressing mix
1   cup fat-free buttermilk
3   Tbsp extra virgin olive oil
3/4 cup fat-free sour cream
1   Tbsp dried dill weed
4   cups prepackaged Romaine lettuce

1. Combine all ingredients except lettuce in a medium bowl and whisk until well blended. Cover with plastic wrap and refrigerate at least 30 minutes to thicken slightly. For peak flavor and texture, refrigerate at least 8 hours.

2. Place mixed greens in a salad bowl, add 1/2 cup of the dressing, and toss, gently yet thoroughly, to coat. Store remaining dressing in refrigerator for later use.

Exchanges

1 Vegetable

1/2 Fat

Calories 49
  Calories from Fat . . . 23
Total Fat . . . . 3 g
  Saturated Fat . . . . 1 g
Cholesterol . . . . 1 mg
Sodium . . . . 174 mg
Total Carbohydrate . . 5 g
  Dietary Fiber . . . . 0 g
  Sugars . . . . 3 g
Protein . . . . 2 g

Baby Spinach and Pasta Salad

If pitted olives are not available, place olives one at a time on a cutting board and press down with the flat side of a butcher knife. That will flatten the olive, releasing the seed easily.

PREPARATION TIME
15 minutes

SERVES
7

SERVING SIZE
1 cup

Exchanges

1/2 Starch

1/2 Fat

Calories 76
 Calories from Fat . . . 21
Total Fat . . . . 2 g
 Saturated Fat . . . . 1 g
Cholesterol . . . . 4 mg
Sodium . . . . 193 mg
Total Carbohydrate . 11 g
 Dietary Fiber . . . . 1 g
 Sugars . . . . 1 g
Protein . . . . 3 g

3 oz uncooked wheat or multi-colored corkscrew pasta (about 1 cup)
3 oz prepackaged spinach leaves, stems removed, preferably baby spinach
2 Tbsp balsamic vinegar
1 1/2 tsp dried oregano or basil
1/4 tsp salt
1/8 tsp black pepper
1 1/2 oz feta cheese with basil and sun-dried tomatoes, crumbled
12 small kalamata or ripe olives

1. Cook pasta according to directions on the package, omitting any salt or fat. Drain and rinse under cold running water to stop cooking process and cool quickly. Shake off excess liquid.
2. Place spinach in a salad bowl and add cooled and drained pasta. Toss with the vinegar, herbs, salt, and pepper. Add feta and olives and toss gently. Serve immediately.

Spring Greens with Raspberry Spice Vinaigrette

It's easy to combine salad dressing ingredients in a jar rather than whisking in a bowl. The dressing blends easily, with less mess and effort … and you can store any unused dressing in same jar.

PREPARATION TIME
15 minutes

SERVES
4

SERVING SIZE
1/4 recipe

1 oz sliced almonds (1/3 cup)
1/4 cup raspberry vinegar
3 Tbsp honey
1/4 tsp ground ginger (optional)
1/4 tsp ground cinnamon
1/4 tsp salt
4 cups prepackaged spring greens
1 cup mandarin oranges or sliced strawberries or blueberries

1. Heat a 12-inch nonstick skillet over medium-high heat. Add almonds and cook 4 minutes or until just beginning to turn golden, stirring frequently. Remove from heat and cool completely.

2. Meanwhile, in a jar, combine vinegar, honey, ginger, cinnamon, and salt. Cover with lid and shake vigorously until well blended.

3. Place greens in a salad bowl, add salad dressing, and toss gently. Top with fruit and almonds and serve immediately.

Exchanges

1 1/2 Carbohydrate
1/2 Fat

Calories 117
   Calories from Fat . . . 35
Total Fat . . . . 4 g
   Saturated Fat . . . . 0 g
Cholesterol . . . . 0 mg
Sodium . . . . 156 mg
Total Carbohydrate . 21 g
   Dietary Fiber . . . . 2 g
   Sugars . . . . 17 g
Protein . . . . 2 g

Shredded Chipotle Taco Salad

Chipotle salsa is easy to find in your supermarket. Just check the front labels of some common salsas.

PREPARATION TIME
5 minutes

SERVES
6

SERVING SIZE
1/6 recipe

4 oz shredded lettuce
3/4 cup canned black beans, rinsed and drained
2/3 cup chipotle salsa
6 Tbsp reduced-fat sour cream
3/4 cup shredded reduced-fat sharp cheddar cheese
2 oz baked tortilla chips, crumbled

In a 9-inch glass pie pan, layer ingredients in order, starting with lettuce and ending with chips.

Exchanges

1 Starch

1 Lean Meat

Calories 131
   Calories from Fat . . . 43
Total Fat . . . . 5 g
   Saturated Fat . . . . . . 2 g
Cholesterol . . . . 15 mg
Sodium . . . . 284 mg
Total Carbohydrate . 16 g
   Dietary Fiber . . . . 4 g
   Sugars . . . . 2 g
Protein . . . . 8 g

Angel Slaw with Orange-Ginger Vinaigrette

Finely shredded or "angel hair" cabbage is available in some supermarkets. If it's not in yours, use regular shredded cabbage.

PREPARATION TIME
3 minutes

SERVES
6

SERVING SIZE
1/2 cup

3 Tbsp frozen orange-pineapple or orange juice concentrate, thawed
1 Tbsp honey
1 1/2 tsp vegetable oil
1 1/2 tsp cider vinegar
1/2 tsp ground ginger
4 cups finely shredded prepackaged cabbage

1. In a small mixing bowl, combine all ingredients except cabbage. Using a fork, stir until well blended.
2. To serve, pour over slaw and toss gently.

Exchanges

1/2 Carbohydrate

Calories 47
   Calories from Fat . . . 12
Total Fat . . . . 1 g
   Saturated Fat . . . . 0 g
Cholesterol . . . . 0 mg
Sodium . . . . 9 mg
Total Carbohydrate . . 9 g
   Dietary Fiber . . . . 1 g
   Sugars . . . . 8 g
Protein . . . . 1 g

Balsamic Asparagus and Hearts of Palm

You may cook, cool, and store this asparagus covered with plastic wrap up to 24 hours in advance. Then assemble your salad when you're ready to serve.

PREPARATION TIME
10 minutes

SERVES
6

SERVING SIZE
1/6 recipe

Exchanges

1 Vegetable

1/2 Fat

Calories 46
   Calories from Fat . . . 22
Total Fat . . . . 2 g
   Saturated Fat . . . . 0 g
Cholesterol . . . . 0 mg
Sodium . . . . 199 mg
Total Carbohydrate . . 5 g
   Dietary Fiber . . . . 2 g
   Sugars . . . . 2 g
Protein . . . . 2 g

1 cup water
12 asparagus spears, trimmed (about 8 oz)
1 14.5-oz can hearts of palm, drained
2 Tbsp balsamic vinegar
1 Tbsp extra virgin olive oil
1 tsp dried oregano
  Dash salt (optional)
  Dash black pepper (optional)
1 2-oz can diced pimiento

1. Prepare a large bowl of ice water.
2. Bring 1 cup water to boil in a 12-inch nonstick skillet. Add asparagus spears in a single layer, cover tightly, reduce heat, and simmer 2–3 minutes or until asparagus is just tender-crisp.
3. Immediately remove asparagus from skillet and immerse in ice water. Let stand 1–2 minutes or until completely cooled. Drain on paper towels and pat dry.
4. Place asparagus on serving platter and arrange hearts of palm on top.
5. In a small jar, combine vinegar, oil, oregano, salt, and pepper and shake well. Pour vinegar mixture evenly over vegetables and sprinkle with pimiento. Serve immediately for peak color and flavor.

Marinated Artichoke and Mushroom-Basil Salad

To clean mushrooms quickly, use a mushroom brush or lightly wipe mushrooms with a damp paper towel.

PREPARATION TIME
10 minutes

SERVES
6

SERVING SIZE
1/6 recipe

Exchanges

1 Vegetable

1/2 Fat

Calories 57

Calories from Fat . . . 23

Total Fat . . . . 3 g

Saturated Fat . . . . 0 g

Cholesterol . . . . 0 mg

Sodium . . . . 220 mg

Total Carbohydrate . . 8 g

Dietary Fiber . . . . 1 g

Sugars . . . . 3 g

Protein . . . . 2 g

1 14-oz can quartered artichoke hearts, drained
8 oz whole mushrooms, preferably small
16 cherry tomatoes, preferably sweet grape variety
1/2 oz fresh basil, torn into small pieces or 1 Tbsp dried basil
3 Tbsp white balsamic vinegar
1 Tbsp extra virgin olive oil
1/4 tsp salt
1/8 tsp black pepper

1. Place all ingredients in a gallon zippered plastic bag, seal tightly, and gently toss back and forth to coat completely.
2. Lay on a flat surface and marinate at least 1 hour, but not more than 4 hours before serving, turning occasionally.

Creamy Pea and Macaroni Salad

You may refrigerate cooled, drained pasta up to 24 hours in advance and assemble your salad when you're ready to serve.

PREPARATION TIME
5 minutes

SERVES
4

SERVING SIZE
1/2 cup

2 oz uncooked elbow macaroni
1 cup frozen green peas, partially thawed
2 Tbsp light mayonnaise
1/2 tsp dried dill weed
1/4 tsp salt
1/8 tsp black pepper

1. Cook pasta according to package directions, omitting any salt or fat.
2. Drain in colander and run under cold tap water until completely cool. Drain extremely well, shaking any excess water from pasta.
3. Place pasta in mixing bowl with remaining ingredients, stir to blend thoroughly, and serve immediately.

Exchanges

1 Starch

1/2 Fat

Calories 109
    Calories from Fat . . . 25
Total Fat . . . . 3 g
    Saturated Fat . . . . 0 g
Cholesterol . . . . 2 mg
Sodium . . . . 241 mg
Total Carbohydrate . 17 g
    Dietary Fiber . . . . 3 g
    Sugars . . . . 3 g
Protein . . . . 4 g

Cold and Creamy Sweet Corn Salad

This salad is great with cold chicken or ham.

2 cups frozen corn kernels
2 Tbsp light mayonnaise
1/2 tsp sugar
1/8 tsp cayenne pepper
1/8 tsp ground black pepper or to taste, preferably coarsely ground
1/8 tsp salt

Combine all ingredients and toss gently. Serve immediately.

Exchanges

1 Starch

1/2 Fat

Calories 93
   Calories from Fat . . . 26
Total Fat . . . . 3 g
   Saturated Fat . . . . 0 g
Cholesterol . . . . 2 mg
Sodium . . . . 140 mg
Total Carbohydrate . 17 g
   Dietary Fiber . . . . 2 g
   Sugars . . . . 2 g
Protein . . . . 2 g

Black-Eyed Pea and Barley Salad

You may refrigerate cooked barley up to 24 hours in advance and assemble your salad when you're ready to serve.

PREPARATION TIME
5 minutes

SERVES
6

SERVING SIZE
1/2 cup

Exchanges

1 Starch

1/2 Fat

Calories 107

Calories from Fat . . . 21

Total Fat . . . . 2 g

Saturated Fat . . . . . . 1 g

Cholesterol . . . . 5 mg

Sodium . . . . 231 mg

Total Carbohydrate . 16 g

Dietary Fiber . . . . . . 4 g

Sugars . . . . 2 g

Protein . . . . 6 g

2 cups water
1/4 cup medium barley
1 14.5-oz can black-eyed peas, rinsed and drained
1 4-oz jar diced pimiento, drained
2 Tbsp cider vinegar
1/2 tsp dried thyme
1/4 tsp hot pepper sauce
1/8 tsp salt
1 1/2 oz blue cheese, crumbled

1. Bring water to boil in medium saucepan. Add barley and return to a boil. Reduce heat and simmer, covered, 30 minutes or until barley is just tender.
2. Drain well. Run under cold tap water to cool completely and drain again.
3. Place barley in medium mixing bowl with black-eyed peas, pimiento, vinegar, thyme, pepper sauce, and salt. Toss well, add cheese, toss very gently, and serve immediately.

Cilantro Black Bean and Rice Salad

This is a great way to use leftover rice.

PREPARATION TIME
10 minutes

SERVES
5

SERVING SIZE
1/2 cup

1/2 cup uncooked white rice
1 1/3 cups water
3/4 cup canned black beans, rinsed and drained
1/4 cup fresh cilantro leaves (pinch leaves off stems)
1/4 cup lime juice (2 medium limes)
1/4 tsp salt
1/8 tsp black pepper
2 Tbsp extra virgin olive oil

1. Cook rice according to package directions, using 1 1/3 cups water and omitting any salt or fats. Cool by placing hot rice on a baking sheet or sheet of foil in a thin layer, about 10 minutes.
2. When completely cooled, place rice in a medium mixing bowl with remaining ingredients, and toss gently, yet thoroughly. Serve immediately.

Exchanges

1 1/2 Starch

1 Fat

Calories 153
  Calories from Fat . . . 46
Total Fat . . . . 5 g
  Saturated Fat . . . . 1 g
Cholesterol . . . . 0 mg
Sodium . . . . 157 mg
Total Carbohydrate . 23 g
  Dietary Fiber . . . . 3 g
  Sugars . . . . 1 g
Protein . . . . 4 g

Couscous Salad with Capers and Olives

If you haven't tried couscous yet, you must! It has a great nutty flavor and wonderful texture.

PREPARATION TIME
5 minutes

SERVES
5

SERVING SIZE
1/2 cup

Exchanges

1 Starch

1/2 Fat

Calories 92
   Calories from Fat . . . 25
Total Fat . . . . 3 g
   Saturated Fat . . . . 0 g
Cholesterol . . . . 0 mg
Sodium . . . . 151 mg
Total Carbohydrate . 14 g
   Dietary Fiber . . . . 1 g
   Sugars . . . . 1 g
Protein . . . . 2 g

3/4 cup water
1/2 cup dried uncooked couscous
  2 Tbsp sliced olives, drained
  2 Tbsp capers, rinsed and drained
  2 Tbsp lemon juice
  2 tsp extra virgin olive oil
3/4 tsp dried oregano
1/8 tsp black pepper

1. In a small saucepan, bring water to a boil, stir in couscous, cover tightly, remove from heat, and let stand 5 minutes.
2. Fluff couscous with a fork. Cool by placing hot couscous on a baking sheet or sheet of foil in a thin layer, about 5 minutes.
3. Meanwhile, in a medium bowl, combine remaining ingredients.
4. When couscous is completely cooled, combine with dressing and toss gently.

Meals Maxed at 4

Just when you thought it couldn't get easier: this chapter contains recipes that use only four ingredients (not counting seasonings) to make the main dish! Some meals need only a salad to make them complete; others may need a side of rice, colorful vegetables, or crusty hot bread. But either way, it can't get much simpler than this.

These recipes come in handy when your time is limited. By using high-flavored ingredients and convenience products that contain several ingredients in one product, such as picante sauce or herb stuffing, the ingredient list can be shortened greatly. When you are creating your own recipes, keep in mind that picante sauce is a multi-purpose item. Because it contains peppers, onions, tomatoes, and seasonings, it can be used practically anywhere a recipe calls for these ingredients, and all in one bottle.

My other trick, reducing ingredients—that is, cooking them down to a more concentrated form over high heat—is a wonderful and easy way to get more intense flavor without adding extra ingredients, fat, or time. Just be sure that you remove any meat or poultry from the dish before you reduce or you will overcook it. You'll love this quick way to make a great sauce!

Skillet Chicken and Stuffing

You can make a quick salad and warm some crusty bread while this chicken is baking.

PREPARATION TIME
10 minutes

SERVES
4

SERVING SIZE
1/4 recipe

4 oz lean pork breakfast sausage
1 cup finely chopped green bell pepper
1 1/2 cups herb-seasoned stuffing
1 cup water
4 4-oz boneless skinless chicken breast halves, rinsed and patted dry
Black pepper to taste
Paprika to taste (optional)

1. Heat oven to 350°F.

2. Heat a 12-inch nonstick skillet over medium-high heat. Add sausage and cook until no longer pink, about 3 minutes, breaking up larger pieces with a spatula. Reduce heat to medium, add peppers to skillet, and cook 4 minutes or until peppers are tender-crisp.

3. Add stuffing and water and stir thoroughly. Remove from heat, top with chicken breasts, and sprinkle with pepper and paprika, if desired.

4. Cover tightly and bake 22–25 minutes or until chicken is no longer pink in center. Remove from oven. Let stand, covered, 5 minutes to develop flavors before serving.

Exchanges

1 Starch

4 Lean Meat

Calories	287
Calories from Fat	62
Total Fat	7 g
Saturated Fat	2 g
Cholesterol	84 mg
Sodium	551 mg
Total Carbohydrate	19 g
Dietary Fiber	2 g
Sugars	2 g
Protein	33 g

Chicken and Vegetables with Onion Sauce

Only one pot to wash for this easy meal!

PREPARATION TIME
5 minutes

SERVES
5

SERVING SIZE
1/5 recipe

5 4-oz boneless skinless chicken breast halves, rinsed and patted dry
1 1-lb bag frozen stewing vegetables
1 10.5-oz can condensed French onion soup

1. Heat Dutch oven over medium-high heat. Coat with cooking spray, add chicken, and top with vegetables and soup. Bring to a boil, cover tightly, reduce heat, and simmer 20 minutes or until carrots are tender.
2. Remove chicken and vegetables with a slotted spoon and place in serving bowl.
3. Increase to high heat, bring pan drippings to a boil and continue boiling one minute or until the liquid measures 1/2 cup. Spoon sauce over chicken and serve.

Exchanges

1 Starch

3 Very Lean Meat

Calories 194

   Calories from Fat . . . 22

Total Fat . . . . 2 g

   Saturated Fat . . . . 0 g

Cholesterol . . . . 65 mg

Sodium . . . . 570 mg

Total Carbohydrate . 12 g

   Dietary Fiber . . . . 2 g

   Sugars . . . . 6 g

Protein . . . . 28 g

Sweet and Tangy Chicken

You'll need to use a coated metal, wooden, or heat-tempered plastic spatula to reduce this sauce rather than a regular plastic spatula.

PREPARATION TIME
5 minutes

SERVES
4

SERVING SIZE
1/4 recipe

Exchanges

1/2 Carbohydrate

4 Very Lean Meat

Calories 167
  Calories from Fat . . . 28
Total Fat . . . . 3 g
  Saturated Fat . . . . 1 g
Cholesterol . . . . 68 mg
Sodium . . . . 467 mg
Total Carbohydrate . . 7 g
  Dietary Fiber . . . . 0 g
  Sugars . . . . 7 g
Protein . . . . 26 g

  2 Tbsp sugar
  2 Tbsp Dijon mustard
1 1/2 Tbsp lite soy sauce
  4 4-oz boneless skinless chicken breast halves, rinsed and patted dry
1/4 cup water

1. In a small bowl, combine sugar, mustard, and soy sauce. Stir to blend thoroughly.
2. Place chicken in a shallow bowl, such as a pie pan. Spoon two Tbsp of the mustard mixture evenly over chicken and turn several times to coat lightly. Let stand 15 minutes.
3. Heat a 12-inch nonstick skillet over medium-high heat. Add chicken and cook 6 minutes. Turn and cook 4 minutes longer or until no longer pink in center. Place chicken on clean plate and set aside.
4. Add reserved mustard mixture and water to the skillet, bring to a boil, and continue boiling 1 1/2 minutes or until sauce is thickened slightly, scraping the bottom of the skillet with a flat spatula. Spoon sauce over chicken to serve.

Beef Sirloin with Onions

Allowing the beef to stand at room temperature for a few minutes "relaxes" it, preventing it from becoming tough over high heat.

PREPARATION TIME
10 minutes

SERVES
4

SERVING SIZE
1/4 recipe

Exchanges

3 Lean Meat

Calories 184	
Calories from Fat. . . 74	
Total Fat. . . . . 8 g	
Saturated Fat. . . . . . . 3 g	
Cholesterol . . . . 54 mg	
Sodium . . . . 417 mg	
Total Carbohydrate . . 4 g	
Dietary Fiber . . . . 1 g	
Sugars . . . . 3 g	
Protein . . . . 22 g	

1   lb sirloin steak, trimmed of fat, cut into 1-inch cubes
2   Tbsp lite soy sauce, divided
1   Tbsp Worcestershire sauce
1/4   tsp black pepper
1   4-oz yellow onion, cut in eighths

1. In a gallon-size zippered plastic bag, combine beef and 1 Tbsp soy sauce, seal tightly, shake to blend, and let stand at room temperature for 15 minutes.
2. In a small bowl, combine remaining soy sauce, Worcestershire sauce, and pepper and set aside.
3. Heat a 12-inch nonstick skillet over high heat. Add beef and cook 1 1/2 minutes or until browned on edges, stirring constantly. Remove beef from skillet and set aside on separate plate.
4. Reduce heat to medium high and add onions to pan drippings. Cook 4 minutes or until just tender-crisp. The layers will separate while cooking.
5. Increase heat to high, add beef and soy mixture to onions, and cook 30 seconds or until richly glazed, stirring constantly (liquid will evaporate). Serve immediately.

Meat Loaf Picante

Put your feet up and watch the news after you slide this incredibly easy meat loaf into the oven!

PREPARATION TIME
5 minutes

SERVES
4

SERVING SIZE
2 slices

1   lb lean ground beef (96% fat-free)
2/3 cup picante sauce, divided
1/3 cup quick-cooking oats
1   egg white
1/8 tsp salt
1/4 tsp black pepper

1. Heat oven to 350°F. Coat a baking rack and pan with cooking spray.
2. In a medium bowl, combine ground beef with 1/3 cup picante sauce, oats, egg white, salt, and pepper. Mix until blended.
3. Shape meat into an oval about 5 inches wide by 7 inches long and 2 inches thick. Place meat loaf on rack and spoon remaining picante sauce evenly over the top.
4. Bake 50 minutes or until no longer pink in center. Remove from oven and let stand 5 minutes for easier slicing. Cut into 8 slices.

Exchanges

1/2 Carbohydrate

4 Very Lean Meat

Calories 185
   Calories from Fat. . . 46
Total Fat. . . . . 5 g
   Saturated Fat. . . . . . . 2 g
Cholesterol . . . . 59 mg
Sodium . . . . 401 mg
Total Carbohydrate . . 7 g
   Dietary Fiber . . . . 1 g
   Sugars . . . . 2 g
Protein . . . . 27 g

Hamburger Roundup

You can use a different shape of pasta in this beefy dish if you prefer.

PREPARATION TIME
4 minutes

SERVES
4

SERVING SIZE
1/4 recipe

Exchanges

1 1/2 Starch

3 Very Lean Meat

1 Vegetable

Calories 272

   Calories from Fat. . . 35

Total Fat. . . . . 4 g

   Saturated Fat. . . . . . . 1 g

Cholesterol . . . . 58 mg

Sodium . . . . 422 mg

Total Carbohydrate . 30 g

   Dietary Fiber . . . . 2 g

   Sugars . . . . 6 g

Protein . . . . 28 g

4 oz uncooked small elbow macaroni
1 lb lean ground beef (96% fat-free)
8 oz frozen pepper-onion stir-fry, thawed
1/3 cup ketchup
1/4 cup pasta water
1/4 tsp salt

1. Cook macaroni according to package directions, omitting any salt or fat.
2. Meanwhile, heat a 12-inch nonstick skillet over high heat. Add beef and cook 3 minutes or until no longer pink. Add stir-fry and cook 3 minutes or until onions are tender, stirring constantly. Stir in ketchup, remove skillet from heat, and cover to keep warm.
3. When macaroni is cooked, add pasta water, drained macaroni, and salt to the beef mixture. Stir and serve.

Thick and Beefy Pinto Bean Stew

Try this stew over rice or noodles, or serve it with coleslaw and warm whole-wheat bread.

PREPARATION TIME
5 minutes

SERVES
4

SERVING SIZE
1/4 recipe

8   oz lean ground beef (96% fat-free)
1   15.5-oz can pinto beans, rinsed and drained
1   14.5-oz can stewed tomatoes, Cajun-style
3/4 cup water
2   tsp ground cumin
1/2 tsp black pepper

1. Heat a large nonstick saucepan over medium-high heat. Add beef and cook 2 minutes or until no longer pink, stirring constantly. Add beans, tomatoes, and water. Bring to a boil, reduce heat, cover tightly, and simmer 15 minutes.
2. Remove from heat and stir in cumin and pepper.

Exchanges

1 1/2 Starch

2 Very Lean Meat

1 Vegetable

Calories	198
Calories from Fat . . .	25
Total Fat	3 g
Saturated Fat	1 g
Cholesterol	29 mg
Sodium	353 mg
Total Carbohydrate .	24 g
Dietary Fiber	8 g
Sugars	6 g
Protein	19 g

Dijon Pork and Roasted Sweet Potato Cubes

Sweet potatoes make this dish unusually pretty.

PREPARATION TIME
15 minutes

SERVES
4

SERVING SIZE
1/4 recipe

Exchanges

1 1/2 Starch

3 Very Lean Meat

1/2 Fat

Calories 255	
Calories from Fat. . . 60	
Total Fat. . . . . 7 g	
Saturated Fat. . . . . . 2 g	
Cholesterol . . . . 65 mg	
Sodium . . . . 326 mg	
Total Carbohydrate . 23 g	
Dietary Fiber . . . . . . 3 g	
Sugars . . . . 11 g	
Protein . . . . 26 g	

1   lb pork tenderloin, trimmed of fat
3   Tbsp Dijon mustard
     Black pepper to taste
1   lb sweet potatoes, peeled and cut
     into bite-size pieces
2   tsp extra virgin olive oil

1. Heat oven to 425°F.
2. Coat pork with mustard evenly, sprinkle liberally with black pepper, and let stand 15 minutes.
3. In a medium bowl, toss potatoes with olive oil and place on outer edges of nonstick baking sheet, allowing space between each piece. Place pork tenderloin in center of baking sheet, tucking thin end under to roast evenly.
4. Bake 10 minutes. Using 2 spoons, stir potatoes and bake 10 minutes longer or until tender. Remove potatoes, cover, and keep warm. Continue cooking pork 5 minutes or until pork is barely pink in center.
5. Remove pork and place on cutting board. Let stand 5 minutes to finish cooking and permit easier slicing. Slice pork in 1/4-inch slices and arrange around potatoes.

Fresh Lime'd Pork

This dish is great with wild rice and asparagus.

PREPARATION TIME
10 minutes

SERVES
4

SERVING SIZE
1/4 recipe

Exchanges

4 Lean Meat

Calories	230
Calories from Fat	121
Total Fat	13 g
Saturated Fat	5 g
Cholesterol	77 mg
Sodium	128 mg
Total Carbohydrate	1 g
Dietary Fiber	0 g
Sugars	0 g
Protein	25 g

1 lb boneless pork chops, cut in thin strips
2 medium limes
1 1/2 tsp grated gingerroot
2 Tbsp chopped fresh cilantro, divided
1/8 tsp salt
Black pepper to taste

1. Place pork in a shallow bowl or pie pan. Squeeze the juice of 1 lime over pork, add ginger and 1 Tbsp of the cilantro, and stir to blend. Let stand at room temperature 15 minutes. Remove pork from marinade and pat dry.
2. Heat a 12-inch nonstick skillet over high heat. Spray skillet with nonstick cooking spray. Add half the pork and cook 2–3 minutes or until beginning to brown, stirring constantly for even cooking. Remove from skillet and place on separate plate. Repeat with remaining pork.
3. Add first batch of pork to second and cook 15 seconds to heat through. Place on serving platter, sprinkle with remaining 1 Tbsp cilantro, and squeeze the juice of the remaining lime evenly over all. Sprinkle with salt and pepper and serve immediately.

Onion Pork Chops

These bone-in pork chops are more economical than their boneless cousins.

PREPARATION TIME
10 minutes

SERVES
4

SERVING SIZE
1/4 recipe

Exchanges

3 Lean Meat

1 Vegetable

Calories 164	
Calories from Fat . . . 54	
Total Fat . . . . 6 g	
Saturated Fat . . . . 2 g	
Cholesterol . . . . 59 mg	
Sodium . . . . 191 mg	
Total Carbohydrate . . 6 g	
Dietary Fiber . . . . 1 g	
Sugars . . . . 4 g	
Protein . . . . 21 g	

4 pork chops with bone in, trimmed of fat (about 5 oz each)
1 medium yellow onion, thinly sliced
2 Tbsp balsamic vinegar, divided
1/4 tsp salt
1/8 tsp black pepper

1. Heat a 12-inch nonstick skillet over high heat. Add pork chops and cook 2 minutes, then remove and set aside on plate.
2. Reduce heat to medium high, add onion, and cook 5 minutes or until richly browned, stirring frequently.
3. Place pork (browned side up) and any accumulated juices on top of onions. Sprinkle with 1 Tbsp of the vinegar, reduce heat, cover tightly, and simmer 8 minutes or until pork is no longer pink in center.
4. Remove pork and onions with slotted spatula and place on a serving platter. Add remaining vinegar to pan drippings, increase heat to high, and cook 1 minute or until liquid measures 1/4 cup. Pour over pork and onions, and sprinkle with salt and pepper to serve.

Rustic Cabbage and Noodles

This German dish is fun to make on a cold winter night.

PREPARATION TIME
20 minutes

SERVES
4

SERVING SIZE
1/4 recipe

Exchanges

2 Starch

2 Vegetable

1 Fat

Calories 269
    Calories from Fat . . . 54
Total Fat . . . . 6 g
    Saturated Fat . . . . . . 2 g
Cholesterol . . . . 7 mg
Sodium . . . . 431 mg
Total Carbohydrate . 43 g
    Dietary Fiber . . . . 6 g
    Sugars . . . . 10 g
Protein . . . . 10 g

6 oz uncooked no-yolk egg noodles
4 bacon slices, cut into very small pieces
6 cups coarsely chopped green cabbage, about 1-inch pieces (do not shred!)
2 cups chopped yellow onions
4 garlic cloves, minced
1/2 tsp salt
   Black pepper to taste

1. Cook noodles according to package directions, omitting any salt or fat.
2. Meanwhile, heat 12-inch skillet over medium heat. Add bacon and cook until very crisp. Drain bacon on paper towels. Drain off excess grease, reserving 2 tsp of the grease.
3. Increase skillet heat to high, add reserved grease, and tilt skillet to coat bottom of pan evenly. Add cabbage, onions, and garlic and cook 4 minutes, tossing **frequently**, using two utensils for easier tossing. Cook an additional 3 minutes, tossing **constantly** or until onions are translucent and beginning to richly brown.
4. Remove from heat and stir in salt, bacon, and pepper. Cover and let stand 3 minutes to develop flavors. Serve over egg noodles.

Peasant-Style White Beans and Rice

Using brown rice instead of white in this recipe will give a heavier, nuttier flavor.

PREPARATION TIME
5 minutes

SERVES
4

SERVING SIZE
1 cup

1   cup uncooked white rice
1   16-oz can navy beans, rinsed and drained
3   Tbsp chopped fresh basil or 1 Tbsp dried basil
2   Tbsp chopped fresh parsley
2   Tbsp extra virgin olive oil
1/2   tsp salt
1   lemon, cut into 8 wedges

1. Cook rice according to package directions, omitting any salt or fat.
2. When rice is cooked, place in pasta bowl. Top with beans, basil, and parsley and toss very gently. Drizzle oil over the top and sprinkle with salt. Serve immediately with lemon wedges.

Exchanges

4 Starch

1/2 Fat

Calories 332
    Calories from Fat. . . 61
Total Fat. . . . . 7 g
    Saturated Fat. . . . . . 1 g
Cholesterol . . . . 0 mg
Sodium . . . . 459 mg
Total Carbohydrate . 57 g
    Dietary Fiber . . . . . . 6 g
    Sugars . . . . 2 g
Protein . . . . 10 g

Feta'd Eggplant with Tomatoes

You can use any shape pasta in this dish ... try vermicelli!

PREPARATION TIME
5 minutes

SERVES
4

SERVING SIZE
1/4 recipe

Exchanges

1 1/2 Starch

3 Vegetable

1 Fat

Calories 232
   Calories from Fat . . . 53
Total Fat . . . . 6 g
   Saturated Fat . . . . 3 g
Cholesterol . . . . 15 mg
Sodium . . . . 564 mg
Total Carbohydrate . 35 g
   Dietary Fiber . . . . 5 g
   Sugars . . . . 11 g
Protein . . . . 10 g

4 oz uncooked penne pasta
1 14.5-oz can diced tomatoes seasoned with peppers and onions
1 lb eggplant, cut in 8 1/4-inch slices
3 oz feta cheese seasoned with sun-dried tomatoes and basil, crumbled

1. Heat broiler.
2. Cook pasta according to package directions, omitting any salt or fat.
3. Pour tomatoes with liquid into a 12-inch nonstick skillet and bring to a boil over high heat. Continue to boil 3 minutes or until most of the liquid has evaporated and remainder measures 1 cup. Remove from heat and set aside.
4. Meanwhile, arrange eggplant slices on a nonstick baking sheet. Lightly spray slices with cooking spray and broil no closer than 5–6 inches away from heat source for 3 minutes. Turn and broil 3 minutes or until lightly brown and tender.
5. Remove from broiler, top each eggplant slice with equal amounts of tomato mixture (about 2 Tbsp per slice), and sprinkle crumbled feta evenly over all. Broil 1 minute longer to heat through and allow cheese to melt slightly. Serve over hot pasta.

Fisherman Oyster Chowder

You can make this chowder with clams if you prefer.

PREPARATION TIME
5 minutes

SERVES
4

SERVING SIZE
1 cup

2 cups finely chopped yellow onion
1 pint oysters with liquid
2 cups fat-free milk
3 Tbsp reduced-fat margarine
1/4 tsp salt
1/4 tsp black pepper

1. Heat a 3-qt nonstick saucepan over medium-high heat. Add onions and cook 8–10 minutes or until translucent. Add oysters and cook 2–3 minutes or until oysters begin to slightly curl on edges.
2. Add milk and cook until thoroughly heated, about 8–10 minutes, stirring occasionally.
3. Remove from heat and stir in margarine, salt, and pepper to serve.

Exchanges

1 Carbohydrate

1 Lean Meat

1 Fat

Calories 189
  Calories from Fat . . . 69
Total Fat . . . . 8 g
  Saturated Fat . . . . 1 g
Cholesterol . . . . 64 mg
Sodium . . . . 394 mg
Total Carbohydrate . 17 g
  Dietary Fiber . . . . 1 g
  Sugars . . . . 15 g
Protein . . . . 13 g

Already Stocked Suppers

No need to stop and pick something up or call for delivery. Keep ingredients on hand for these "already stocked" suppers, ideal after a long day when you just want to get home—but don't want to starve when you get there!

Now you'll never be lost for dinner ideas ... or be able to say, "but there's nothing in the house!" Try keeping these basics on hand and you'll be surprised at the peace of mind it brings you, knowing you can always whip up a quick, healthy meal. You can easily thaw any frozen pound of meat or poultry in 8 minutes in the microwave and you're ready to go!

Or try adding your favorite marinade to meat or poultry when you bring it home from the supermarket. Just drop the meat or poultry in a freezer zippered bag along with the marinade, seal it tightly (releasing any excess air), and freeze for later use. The meat marinates for just the right amount of time as it slowly freezes. Then just defrost and use. It's an easy way to add flavor and variety to frozen meat.

Rosemary Chicken with Oven-Roasted Potatoes

Some people like the extra lemony flavor added by the zest, but just omit it for more delicate palates.

PREPARATION TIME
5 minutes

SERVES
4

SERVING SIZE
1/4 recipe

Exchanges

1 1/2 Starch

4 Very Lean Meat

Calories 245	
Calories from Fat . . . 29	
Total Fat . . . . 3 g	
Saturated Fat . . . . 1 g	
Cholesterol . . . . 78 mg	
Sodium . . . . 223 mg	
Total Carbohydrate . 21 g	
Dietary Fiber . . . . 2 g	
Sugars . . . . 2 g	
Protein . . . . 31 g	

4	8-oz chicken breasts with bone in and skin on, rinsed and patted dry (2 lb)
1/2	tsp grated lemon zest (optional)
2	Tbsp lemon juice
1/4	tsp dried rosemary
8	2-oz new potatoes, halved crosswise
	Paprika to taste
1/4	tsp salt
1	medium lemon, cut into eight wedges

1. Heat oven to 400°F.
2. Arrange chicken breasts on a nonstick baking sheet. Pull skin back without detaching completely.
3. Sprinkle lemon zest, lemon juice, and rosemary under skin; replace skin over breasts and arrange potatoes around chicken.
4. Lightly coat chicken with cooking spray, sprinkle with paprika, and bake 45 minutes or until chicken is no longer pink in center and potatoes are tender.
5. Remove from oven, discard skin, place potatoes and chicken on serving platter, and sprinkle salt evenly over all. Serve with lemon wedges.

Mozzarella and Green Chili Chicken

To flatten chicken easily, place chicken breasts about 2 inches apart on a sheet of plastic wrap about 18 inches long. Top with another sheet of plastic wrap the same length. Using the flat side of a meat mallet or the bottom of a bottle, flatten chicken breasts until they are 1/4-inch thick. Flattening the chicken will make it easier to wrap around the cheese stick and will help it cook evenly.

PREPARATION TIME
15 minutes

SERVES
4

SERVING SIZE
1/4 recipe

Exchanges

2 Starch

3 Lean Meat

Calories 331

   Calories from Fat. . . 71

Total Fat. . . . . 8 g

   Saturated Fat. . . . . . 4 g

Cholesterol . . . . 82 mg

Sodium . . . . 456 mg

Total Carbohydrate . 28 g

   Dietary Fiber . . . . . . 2 g

   Sugars . . . . 0 g

Protein . . . . 33 g

3/4 cup uncooked brown or white rice
1 1/2 cups water
4 4-oz boneless, skinless chicken breast halves, rinsed and patted dry and flattened to 1/4-inch thickness
1 4-oz can chopped mild green chilis
4 3/4-oz Mozzarella cheese sticks
3/4 tsp ground cumin
1/8 tsp salt
  Black pepper to taste
1 medium lime, cut into eight wedges

1. Heat oven to 400°F.
2. Cook rice according to package directions using 1 1/2 cups water, omitting any salt or fat.
3. Meanwhile, coat an 8-inch by 12-inch baking dish with cooking spray and arrange chicken pieces smooth side down.
4. Spoon 2 Tbsp green chilis onto each chicken breast. Using the back of the spoon, spread evenly to coat each breast. Place a cheese stick in the center of each piece of chicken and fold in sides, overlapping slightly. Place seam side down in baking dish. Sprinkle evenly with cumin, salt, and pepper.
5. Bake, uncovered, for 18 minutes or until chicken is no longer pink in center.
6. Place rice on serving platter and top with chicken and any accumulated juices. Serve with lime wedges.

Orange-Ginger Steakhouse Sirloin

This sauce is surprisingly good on salmon, too.

PREPARATION TIME
5 minutes

SERVES
5

SERVING SIZE
1/5 recipe

Exchanges

3 Lean Meat

Calories 154	
Calories from Fat . . . 44	
Total Fat . . . . 5 g	
Saturated Fat . . . . 2 g	
Cholesterol . . . . 64 mg	
Sodium . . . . 199 mg	
Total Carbohydrate . . 3 g	
Dietary Fiber . . . . 0 g	
Sugars . . . . 3 g	
Protein . . . . 22 g	

1/4 cup steak sauce
  1 Tbsp sugar
  1 tsp orange zest
1/2 tsp ground ginger
  1 20-oz boneless sirloin steak, about
     3/4 inch thick, trimmed of fat
     (20 oz after trimming)

1. Heat broiler.
2. In a small bowl, combine steak sauce, sugar, orange zest, and ginger. Place beef in a shallow baking dish and spoon all but 2 Tbsp steak sauce mixture over steak. Turn several times to coat thoroughly. Let stand at room temperature 20 minutes.
3. Coat a broiler rack and pan with cooking spray and place beef on broiler rack, discarding marinade. Broil no closer than 2–3 inches away from heat source for 5 minutes, then turn and broil 4–5 more minutes or until desired doneness.
4. Place on cutting board and let rest 5 minutes before slicing in thin diagonals. Spoon reserved sauce over slices and serve.

Skillet Ground Beef and Corn

Adding salt at the end of the cooking process gives a more pronounced flavor, which means you can use less.

PREPARATION TIME
3 minutes

SERVES
4

SERVING SIZE
1/4 recipe

Exchanges

2 Starch

3 Lean Meat

Calories 309	
Calories from Fat . . . 57	
Total Fat . . . . 6 g	
Saturated Fat . . . . 2 g	
Cholesterol . . . . 87 mg	
Sodium . . . . 523 mg	
Total Carbohydrate . 33 g	
Dietary Fiber . . . . 2 g	
Sugars . . . . 4 g	
Protein . . . . 31 g	

4 oz uncooked no-yolk or whole-wheat egg noodles
1 lb lean ground beef (96% fat-free)
1 cup frozen corn kernels
1 cup water
3/4 cup picante sauce
1 Tbsp chili powder
1/8 tsp salt

1. Cook noodles according to package directions, omitting any salt or fat.
2. Meanwhile, heat a 12-inch nonstick skillet over high heat. Add beef and cook 3 minutes or until no longer pink, stirring constantly. Add corn, picante sauce, water, and chili powder.
3. Bring to a boil, reduce heat, and simmer, uncovered, 10 minutes or until thickened and most of the liquid has been absorbed.
4. Remove from heat, stir in salt, and serve over cooked noodles.

Onion Pork Chops, p. 44
Cheddar'd Yellow Squash, p. 88
Honey Roasted Carrot Wheels and Onions, p. 86

Mozzarella and Green Chili Chicken, p. 52
Free Veggie Stir-Fry, p. 90

Vegetable Macaroni and Cheese, p. 70

Rustic Apple Crisp, p. 104

Cheater's Spaghetti

You'll be amazed how a few quick additions enhances the flavor of bottled spaghetti sauce.

PREPARATION TIME
3 minutes

SERVES
4

SERVING SIZE
1/4 recipe

8 oz uncooked spaghetti, preferably whole wheat
8 oz lean ground beef (96% fat-free)
1/2 cup chopped onion
4 cloves garlic, minced
1 1/2 cups bottled spaghetti sauce
2 Tbsp dried basil
2 Tbsp Parmesan cheese (optional)

1. Cook pasta according to package directions, omitting any salt or fat.
2. Meanwhile, heat a nonstick saucepan over medium-high heat. Cook beef, onion, and garlic until onion is translucent, stirring frequently. Stir in spaghetti sauce and basil.
3. Bring to a boil, reduce heat, cover tightly, and simmer 10 minutes. Spoon over pasta and top with cheese, if desired.

Exchanges

3 Starch

2 Lean Meat

2 Vegetable

Calories 389

  Calories from Fat . . . 70

Total Fat . . . . 8 g

  Saturated Fat . . . . 2 g

Cholesterol . . . . 29 mg

Sodium . . . . 496 mg

Total Carbohydrate . 59 g

  Dietary Fiber . . . . 5 g

  Sugars . . . . 5 g

Protein . . . . 21 g

Family-Style Vegetable Beef Soup

This soup freezes well. Try freezing it in 1-cup servings so you can pop it in the microwave for a quick lunch.

PREPARATION TIME
8 minutes

SERVES
9

SERVING SIZE
1 cup

1   lb lean ground beef (96% fat-free)
2   14.5-oz cans stewed tomatoes
2   cups fresh or frozen diced green bell peppers
1   10-oz pkg frozen mixed vegetables
2   cups water
1   Tbsp Worcestershire sauce
3   Tbsp ketchup
1/2 tsp salt
1/4 tsp black pepper

1. Heat a Dutch oven over high heat. Add beef and cook 2 minutes or until no longer pink, stirring constantly. Add tomatoes, peppers, mixed vegetables, water, and Worcestershire.
2. Bring to a boil, reduce heat, cover tightly, and simmer 20 minutes.
3. Remove from heat, stir in ketchup, salt, and pepper and let stand 5 minutes, uncovered, to develop flavors.

Exchanges

1 Carbohydrate

1 Lean Meat

Calories 132
   Calories from Fat . . . 27
Total Fat . . . . 3 g
   Saturated Fat . . . . 1 g
Cholesterol . . . . 34 mg
Sodium . . . . 490 mg
Total Carbohydrate . 14 g
   Dietary Fiber . . . . 2 g
   Sugars . . . . 5 g
Protein . . . . 14 g

Tender Country Pork Chops

Serve these pork chops with noodles, rice, or mashed potatoes.

PREPARATION TIME
5 minutes

SERVES
4

SERVING SIZE
1/4 recipe

1/4 cup flour
1/2 tsp garlic powder
1/2 tsp paprika
1/4 tsp salt
     Black pepper to taste
  4 4-oz boneless pork chops, about
     1/2-inch thick
  2 tsp vegetable oil

1. In a shallow dish, such as a pie pan, combine flour, garlic powder, paprika, salt, and pepper. Stir to blend thoroughly. Coat pork evenly with flour mixture and place on a separate plate.
2. Heat oil in a 12-inch nonstick skillet over medium heat. Add pork and cook 6 minutes, then turn and cook 6 minutes longer or until no longer pink in center.

Exchanges

1/2 Starch

3 Medium-Fat Meat

Calories 278
   Calories from Fat. . 143
Total Fat. . . . . 16 g
   Saturated Fat. . . . . . . 5 g
Cholesterol . . . . 77 mg
Sodium . . . . 197 mg
Total Carbohydrate . . 6 g
   Dietary Fiber . . . . 0 g
   Sugars . . . . 0 g
Protein . . . . 26 g

Creamy Ham and Vegetable Chowder

For a meatless dish, substitute 4 oz chopped pimiento or red bell pepper for the ham.

PREPARATION TIME
15 minutes

SERVES
5

SERVING SIZE
1/5 recipe

Exchanges

2 Carbohydrate

1 Lean Meat

Calories 203
   Calories from Fat. . . 31
Total Fat . . . . 3 g
   Saturated Fat . . . . . . 2 g
Cholesterol . . . . 19 mg
Sodium . . . . 758 mg
Total Carbohydrate . 29 g
   Dietary Fiber . . . . 3 g
   Sugars . . . . 13 g
Protein . . . . 15 g

4   oz extra lean, reduced-sodium ham, thinly sliced and chopped
1   cup water, divided
3/4 cup chopped yellow onion
1   12-oz can evaporated fat-free milk
1   10-oz pkg frozen mixed vegetables, thawed
1   cup potatoes, diced
4   slices reduced-fat American cheese, about 3 oz
1/4 cup reduced-fat sour cream (optional)
1/4 tsp salt
    Black pepper to taste

1. Heat a 2-quart nonstick saucepan over medium-high heat. Add ham and cook 4 minutes or until edges are beginning to lightly brown, stirring frequently. Remove ham from pan and set aside on separate plate.

2. To pan residue, add 1/4 cup water and onion and cook 4 minutes or until onions are translucent. Increase to high heat, add remaining 3/4 cup water and milk and bring just to a boil, stirring frequently. Add mixed vegetables and potatoes and return to a boil, stirring frequently. Reduce heat, cover tightly, and simmer 10 minutes or until potatoes are tender.

3. Using a whisk, stir mixture to break up potatoes and thicken the chowder. Remove from heat and stir in ham and cheese. Cover and let stand 5 minutes to develop flavors. Stir in sour cream, if desired, and salt. Sprinkle with black pepper and serve.

Chunky Kalamata Olive Tomato Sauce

Serve over cooked pasta or spoon over baked chicken or grilled fish.

PREPARATION TIME
10 minutes

SERVES
5

SERVING SIZE
1/2 cup

1 cup finely chopped yellow onions
4 cloves garlic, minced
1 14.5-oz can tomatoes with green bell peppers, celery, and onions, drained (reserve 1/4 cup liquid)
1 cup chopped roasted red peppers
1–2 Tbsp dried basil
16 pitted kalamata olives, coarsely chopped
1/4 tsp salt (optional)

1. Heat medium saucepan over medium-high heat. Coat pan with cooking spray, add onions, and cook 3 minutes or until translucent, stirring frequently. Add garlic and cook 15 seconds longer, stirring constantly. Add tomatoes, the reserved liquid, peppers, and basil.
2. Bring to a boil, reduce heat, and simmer, uncovered, 15 minutes or until onions are tender and most of the liquid has evaporated, stirring occasionally.
3. Remove from heat, stir in olives and salt, cover, and let stand 5 minutes to develop flavors.

Exchanges

2 Vegetable
1/2 Fat

Calories 65
   Calories from Fat . . . 15
Total Fat . . . . 2 g
   Saturated Fat . . . . 0 g
Cholesterol . . . . 0 mg
Sodium . . . . 530 mg
Total Carbohydrate . 12 g
   Dietary Fiber . . . . 3 g
   Sugars . . . . 9 g
Protein . . . . 2 g

Spinach and Artichoke Crustless Tart

To thaw spinach easily, place spinach in its box on a microwaveable plate and microwave on HIGH setting for 3 1/2 minutes or until thawed.

PREPARATION TIME
10 minutes

SERVES
6

SERVING SIZE
1/6 recipe

Exchanges

1 Medium-Fat Meat

1 Vegetable

Calories 106

   Calories from Fat . . . 30

Total Fat . . . . 3 g

   Saturated Fat . . . . 2 g

Cholesterol . . . . 10 mg

Sodium . . . . 452 mg

Total Carbohydrate . . 8 g

   Dietary Fiber . . . . 2 g

   Sugars . . . . 2 g

Protein . . . . 13 g

1 1/2 cups egg substitute (equal to 6 eggs)
  1/3 cup evaporated fat-free milk
    1 10-oz carton frozen chopped
      spinach, thawed and squeezed dry
 1–2 Tbsp dried basil
  1/8 tsp black pepper
    1 14.5-oz can artichoke quarters,
      drained and coarsely chopped
  1/8 tsp salt
    3 oz shredded reduced-fat sharp
      cheddar cheese (3/4 cup)

1. Heat oven to 350°F.
2. Coat a deep-dish pie pan with cooking spray. In pie pan, combine egg substitute, milk, spinach, basil, and black pepper and stir until well blended. Gently stir in artichokes.
3. Bake, uncovered, for 30 minutes. Remove from oven, sprinkle with salt, top with cheese, and let stand 5 minutes to allow flavors to develop and cheese to melt.

Cheesy Corn and Skillet-Roasted Pepper Soup

Exchanges

1 1/2 Carbohydrate

1 Lean Meat

Calories 180	
Calories from Fat . . . 48	
Total Fat . . . . 5 g	
Saturated Fat . . . . . . 3 g	
Cholesterol . . . . 16 mg	
Sodium . . . . 596 mg	
Total Carbohydrate . 24 g	
Dietary Fiber . . . . 3 g	
Sugars . . . . 10 g	
Protein . . . . 12 g	

1 cup chopped yellow onion
2 medium green bell peppers, chopped or 2 cups frozen, diced green peppers, thawed
1 10-oz pkg frozen corn kernels, thawed
1 reduced-sodium chicken bouillon cube
1 1/2 cups water
1 cup evaporated fat-free milk
1 cup shredded reduced-fat sharp cheddar cheese
1/2 tsp salt
1/4 tsp black pepper
1/8 tsp cayenne pepper (optional)

1. Heat a Dutch oven over medium-high heat. Coat Dutch oven with cooking spray, add onion and peppers, and cook 8 minutes or until onions are translucent and beginning to turn golden, stirring frequently.
2. Increase to high heat and add corn, bouillon, and water. Bring to a boil, reduce heat, cover tightly, and simmer 10 minutes.
3. Remove from heat and stir in remaining ingredients.
4. For a thicker consistency, puree half of the mixture by placing one cup in a blender, covering tightly, holding down the lid, and blending until smooth. Repeat once or twice to desired consistency.

Cayenne Fish

Spraying the filets with cooking spray before sprinkling with chili powder helps the chili powder spread slightly, giving the filets good color.

PREPARATION TIME
10 minutes

SERVES
4

SERVING SIZE
1/4 recipe

Exchanges

1 Starch

3 Very Lean Meat

1/2 Fat

Calories 204

Calories from Fat . . . 40

Total Fat . . . . 4 g

Saturated Fat . . . . 0 g

Cholesterol . . . . 59 mg

Sodium . . . . 489 mg

Total Carbohydrate . 17 g

Dietary Fiber . . . . 2 g

Sugars . . . . 2 g

Protein . . . . 23 g

2 cups water
1 2-oz red potato, diced
4 4-oz lean mild fish filets, such as flounder, rinsed and patted dry
1/2 tsp chili powder
2 Tbsp reduced-fat margarine
2 tsp Dijon mustard
1/8 tsp cayenne pepper
1/2 tsp salt
Black pepper to taste

1. Heat oven to 400°F.
2. Place 2 cups water in a large saucepan, place a collapsible steamer basket on bottom of pan, arrange potatoes evenly in basket, and cover tightly. Bring water to a boil and steam potatoes 8 minutes or until just tender.
3. Meanwhile, arrange fish filets on a nonstick baking sheet and lightly coat with cooking spray. Sprinkle evenly with chili powder. Bake fish 10 minutes or until opaque in center.
4. In a small bowl, combine margarine, mustard, cayenne and 1/4 tsp of the salt. Remove potatoes from steamer basket. Take filets out of oven and top with equal amounts of the butter mixture (about 2 tsp per filet). Sprinkle the remaining 1/4 tsp salt and black pepper over potatoes and serve.

Golden Fried Fish

Be sure to rinse and pat the fish dry first. This will allow the dressing and crackers to adhere properly. The oil must be heated before adding the fish or the fish will soak up the oil too quickly and not cook properly.

PREPARATION TIME
10 minutes

SERVES
4

SERVING SIZE
1/4 recipe

Exchanges

1 Starch

3 Lean Meat

Calories 256
   Calories from Fat . . . 92
Total Fat . . . . 10 g
   Saturated Fat . . . . 0 g
Cholesterol . . . . 37 mg
Sodium . . . . 379 mg
Total Carbohydrate . 14 g
   Dietary Fiber . . . . 1 g
   Sugars . . . . 2 g
Protein . . . . 25 g

- 3 Tbsp fat-free Italian salad dressing
- 20 fat-free crackers, coarsely crushed
- 2 tsp paprika
- 1/8 tsp black pepper
- 2 Tbsp vegetable oil
- 4 4-oz lean mild fish filets, such as grouper, rinsed and patted dry
- 1 medium lemon, cut into eight wedges

1. Heat oven to 450°F.

2. Place salad dressing in a shallow dish, such as a pie pan. In another shallow dish or dinner plate, combine cracker crumbs, paprika, and black pepper and stir well to blend thoroughly.

3. Coat a 9-inch by 13-inch baking dish with cooking spray and add oil. Using fingertips, spread oil evenly over bottom of pan. Place dish in oven for 3 minutes.

4. Meanwhile, working quickly and with one filet at a time, coat filet with dressing and then coat with cracker mixture. Place on a clean dinner plate and repeat with remaining filets.

5. When all filets are coated, place in heated baking dish and bake 4 minutes. Carefully turn with a flat spatula and cook 2 minutes longer or until fish is opaque in center. Serve immediately with lemon wedges.

Dump and Do Dinners

When you can't stand the idea of standing over the stove for more than five minutes, it's time to turn to the Dump and Dos. You cook everything at one time in one pot or pan or quickly top an ordinary dish with something delicious. These recipes take a minimal amount of attention, freeing you to clean up quickly, set the table, or simply sit down and relax for a few minutes.

When working in the kitchen, try to think of ways that you can cut corners or combine steps. For instance, cook pasta according to the package directions, but dump the vegetables, such as broccoli, into the pot during the last 5 minutes of the cooking time. This means you only have one pot to wash instead of two. If you are adding canned beans to a pasta dish and want to rinse them first, dump the beans in a colander and drain the cooked pasta over them. This rinses the beans and heats them up at the same time . . . hence, dump and do.

Creamy Chicken and Potatoes

You can also make this dish with pork chops and cream of mushroom soup.

PREPARATION TIME
10 minutes

SERVES
4

SERVING SIZE
1/4 recipe

Exchanges

2 Starch

3 Very Lean Meat

1 Fat

Calories 314

   Calories from Fat . . . 63

Total Fat . . . . 7 g

   Saturated Fat . . . . 3 g

Cholesterol . . . . 85 mg

Sodium . . . . 391 mg

Total Carbohydrate . 30 g

   Dietary Fiber . . . . 3 g

   Sugars . . . . 5 g

Protein . . . . 31 g

1 10-oz can reduced-fat cream of chicken soup
1/2 cup reduced-fat sour cream
4 medium green onions, chopped
4 4-oz boneless skinless chicken breast halves, rinsed and patted dry
1 lb new potatoes, cut into 1/2-inch wedges
  Coarsely ground black pepper

1. In a medium mixing bowl, combine the soup, sour cream and all but 2 Tbsp of the onions and set aside.

2. Heat a 12-inch nonstick skillet over medium-high heat. Add chicken, smooth side down, and cook 1–2 minutes or until lightly browned. Turn pieces over, add potatoes, and pour soup mixture evenly over all.

3. Bring to a boil, reduce heat, cover tightly, and simmer 30 minutes or until chicken is no longer pink in center and potatoes are tender, stirring midway. Top with remaining green onions to serve.

Mexican Drumsticks

To remove the skin from the drumsticks easily, use one paper towel per drumstick. Grasp the skin with the paper towel and pull.

PREPARATION TIME
10 minutes

SERVES
4

SERVING SIZE
1/4 recipe

Exchanges

3 Lean Meat

2 Vegetable

Calories 197
   Calories from Fat . . . 50
Total Fat . . . . 6 g
   Saturated Fat . . . . 1 g
Cholesterol . . . . 78 mg
Sodium . . . . 443 mg
Total Carbohydrate . 11 g
   Dietary Fiber . . . . 2 g
   Sugars . . . . 8 g
Protein . . . . 26 g

  1 14.5-oz can diced tomatoes
1/2 cup chopped yellow onion
3–4 garlic cloves, split in half
  1 Tbsp chili powder
  1 tsp ground cumin
1 1/2 tsp sugar
  8 chicken drumsticks, skin removed
  1 Tbsp lime juice
1/4 tsp salt

1. In a medium mixing bowl, combine tomatoes, onion, garlic, chili powder, cumin, and sugar and set aside.
2. Heat a Dutch oven over high heat. Add chicken and tomato mixture. Bring to a boil, reduce heat, cover tightly, and simmer 45 minutes or until chicken begins to fall off the bone.
3. Place chicken in shallow serving bowl. Add lime juice and salt to tomato mixture and stir, then spoon over chicken.

Chicken with Onion'd Mushrooms

If you can find reduced-sodium onion soup mix, use it!

PREPARATION TIME
5 minutes

SERVES
5

SERVING SIZE
1/5 recipe

1	cup uncooked brown rice
2 1/2	cups water, divided
5	4-oz boneless skinless chicken breast halves, rinsed and patted dry
1	8-oz pkg sliced mushrooms
1	1-oz pkg dried onion soup mix
1	Tbsp balsamic vinegar

1. In a 1-quart saucepan, cook rice according to package directions, using 2 cups water and omitting any salt or fat.
2. Meanwhile, heat a 12-inch nonstick skillet over high heat. Add the chicken, 1/2 cup water, mushrooms, soup mix, and vinegar.
3. Bring to a boil, cover tightly, reduce heat, and simmer 20–22 minutes or until chicken is no longer pink in center. Serve over cooked rice.

Exchanges

2 1/2 Starch

3 Very Lean Meat

Calories 293
   Calories from Fat . . . 29
Total Fat . . . . 3 g
   Saturated Fat . . . . . . 1 g
Cholesterol . . . . 64 mg
Sodium . . . . 621 mg
Total Carbohydrate . 35 g
   Dietary Fiber . . . . 2 g
   Sugars . . . . 4 g
Protein . . . . 31 g

Vegetable Macaroni and Cheese

To thaw vegetables easily, place broccoli mixture and peppers in a colander and run under tap water about 15 seconds, then drain well before continuing with recipe instructions.

PREPARATION TIME
10 minutes

SERVES
7

SERVING SIZE
1 cup

Exchanges

1 1/2 Starch

2 Very Lean Meat

1/2 Fat

Calories 204

   Calories from Fat . . . 38

Total Fat . . . . 4 g

   Saturated Fat . . . . 1 g

Cholesterol . . . . 35 mg

Sodium . . . . 391 mg

Total Carbohydrate . 23 g

   Dietary Fiber . . . . 2 g

   Sugars . . . . 4 g

Protein . . . . 18 g

1   7.25-oz box macaroni and cheese dinner
8   oz frozen broccoli and cauliflower mixture, thawed
4   oz frozen red pepper stir-fry, thawed or 4-oz container sliced pimiento
1/4   cup evaporated fat-free milk
2   Tbsp reduced-fat margarine
9   oz frozen cooked, diced chicken breast meat, thawed (according to package directions)
1/2   tsp salt

1. Cook pasta in boiling water, omitting any salt and fat, for 6 minutes or until almost tender. Add broccoli mixture and peppers to pasta, return to a boil, and boil 2 minutes or until vegetables are just tender-crisp.

2. Drain pasta and vegetables and return to pot. Add cheese mix, milk, and margarine and stir until just blended, using a rubber spatula. Add chicken and salt and stir to blend thoroughly. Serve immediately.

Pizza Mounds

This is a fun way to make pizza, and there's no cutting involved at the end.

PREPARATION TIME
5 minutes

SERVES
4

SERVING SIZE
1/4 recipe

2 whole-wheat pita breads
1/2 cup bottled pizza sauce
(may use spaghetti sauce instead)
4 oz sliced mushrooms
1 tsp dried basil
1 1/2 oz red onion, thinly sliced
3 oz shredded part-skim Mozzarella
cheese (3/4 cup)

1. Heat oven to 400°F.
2. Using a serrated knife, cut each pita in half, creating 4 thin rounds like individual pizzas.
3. Top each round with 1/4 of the ingredients in the order listed.
4. Bake 7 minutes or until edges are lightly golden.

Exchanges

1 Starch

1 Medium-Fat Meat

1 Vegetable

Calories 184
 Calories from Fat . . . 50
Total Fat . . . . 6 g
 Saturated Fat . . . . 3 g
Cholesterol . . . . 16 mg
Sodium . . . . 530 mg
Total Carbohydrate . 22 g
 Dietary Fiber . . . . 1 g
 Sugars . . . . 3 g
Protein . . . . 11 g

Cheddary Ham and Rice Casserole

Get preweighed, thinly sliced ham from the deli so all you have to do is chop it when you get home.

PREPARATION TIME
10 minutes

SERVES
5

SERVING SIZE
1 cup

2 cups water
1 cup uncooked brown or white rice
1 cup finely chopped yellow onion
1/2 cup finely chopped green bell pepper
1/2 cup frozen green peas, thawed
4 oz extra lean, reduced-sodium ham, thinly sliced and chopped
1/4 cup chopped fresh parsley
3 oz shredded reduced-fat cheddar cheese (3/4 cup)
1/2 tsp salt
1/8 tsp cayenne
Black pepper to taste

1. Bring water to a boil in a medium saucepan. Add rice, onion, and bell pepper. Stir, cover, lower heat, and cook for 20 minutes.
2. Remove rice from heat, stir in remaining ingredients, cover, and let stand 3 minutes to allow flavors to develop and cheese to melt.

Exchanges

2 Starch

1 Lean Meat

Calories 226
   Calories from Fat . . . 50
Total Fat . . . . 6 g
   Saturated Fat . . . . 3 g
Cholesterol . . . . 23 mg
Sodium . . . . 658 mg
Total Carbohydrate . 33 g
   Dietary Fiber . . . . 2 g
   Sugars . . . . 4 g
Protein . . . . 11 g

Cheesy Potato and Egg Casserole

To thaw vegetables easily, place peppers and corn in a colander and run under running tap water for 15 seconds, then drain well before continuing with recipe instructions.

PREPARATION TIME
10 minutes

SERVES
6

SERVING SIZE
1/6 recipe

Exchanges

2 Starch

1 Lean Meat

Calories 209
   Calories from Fat . . . 50
Total Fat . . . . 6 g
   Saturated Fat . . . . 3 g
Cholesterol . . . . 23 mg
Sodium . . . . 662 mg
Total Carbohydrate . 27 g
   Dietary Fiber . . . . 4 g
   Sugars . . . . 5 g
Protein . . . . 14 g

1 20-oz pkg refrigerated hash brown potatoes, Southwestern seasoning
1 1/2 cups frozen green bell pepper, thawed
1 cup frozen corn kernels, thawed
4 oz lean, reduced-sodium ham, thinly sliced and chopped
1/2 cup egg substitute
1/3 cup evaporated fat-free milk
1/4 tsp cayenne pepper
1 cup shredded reduced-fat sharp cheddar cheese

1. Heat oven to 350°F.
2. Coat a 12-inch ovenproof skillet with cooking spray and add potatoes, peppers, corn and ham. Pour egg substitute and milk over all and sprinkle with cayenne.
3. Cover and bake 35 minutes or until knife inserted in center comes out clean.
4. Remove from oven, top with cheese, and let stand, uncovered, 3 minutes or until cheese melts.

Mediterranean Ragout

This dish is great served as a stew or over pasta and topped with Parmesan cheese.

Exchanges

1 Carbohydrate

Calories 95	
Calories from Fat . . . 16	
Total Fat . . . . 2 g	
Saturated Fat . . . . 0 g	
Cholesterol . . . . 0 mg	
Sodium . . . . 794 mg	
Total Carbohydrate . 18 g	
Dietary Fiber . . . . 3 g	
Sugars . . . . 10 g	
Protein . . . . 4 g	

8 oz eggplant, diced
8 oz pkg whole mushrooms, wiped clean with damp cloth
1 large green bell pepper, chopped or 7-oz zucchini, sliced
1 14.5-oz can diced tomatoes seasoned with basil, oregano, and garlic, with juice
1/2 cup water
1 tsp dried Italian seasoning
12 pitted kalamata olives, coarsely chopped
1/4 tsp salt

1. Heat a Dutch oven over high heat. Coat with cooking spray and add eggplant, mushrooms, and peppers. Cook 1 minute, then reduce heat to medium high and cook 4 minutes or until eggplant is limp and lightly golden, stirring frequently.
2. Add tomatoes, water, and Italian seasoning, bring to a boil, reduce heat, cover tightly, and simmer 10 minutes.
3. Remove from heat, stir in olives and salt, cover, and let stand 5 minutes.

Veggie Quesadillas

You can serve these with salsa and light sour cream on the side.

PREPARATION TIME
10 minutes

SERVES
4

SERVING SIZE
1/4 recipe

1 4.5-oz can chopped mild green chilis
4 8-inch fat-free flour tortillas
1 6-oz tomato, diced (about 1 cup)
1/2 cup finely chopped green onion
1 cup finely shredded reduced-fat
   sharp cheddar cheese
1/2 tsp ground cumin

1. Heat oven to warm.
2. Spread 2 Tbsp of the chilis on one half of each tortilla. Top green chilis with 1/4 cup of the tomatoes, 2 Tbsp green onion, and 1/4 cup cheese per tortilla. Sprinkle cumin evenly over each tortilla. Fold each tortilla in half and press down gently to adhere.
3. Heat a 12-inch nonstick skillet over medium heat. Add 2 of the tortillas and cook 3 minutes, then turn and cook 2 minutes longer or until cheese has melted. Place on a separate plate in oven to keep warm. Repeat process.
4. Cut each quesadilla in half, starting at the folded edge for easier slicing.

Exchanges

1 1/2 Starch

1 Medium-Fat Meat

1 Vegetable

Calories 204
   Calories from Fat . . . 56
Total Fat . . . . 6 g
   Saturated Fat . . . . 4 g
Cholesterol . . . . 20 mg
Sodium . . . . 714 mg
Total Carbohydrate . 28 g
   Dietary Fiber . . . . 3 g
   Sugars . . . . 2 g
Protein . . . . 12 g

Almond Fish

Try this fish with quick-cooking rice pilaf and coleslaw.

PREPARATION TIME
5 minutes

SERVES
4

SERVING SIZE
1/4 recipe

Exchanges

3 Very Lean Meat

1 Fat

Calories 174
   Calories from Fat. . . 71
Total Fat . . . . 8 g
   Saturated Fat . . . . 0 g
Cholesterol . . . . 60 mg
Sodium . . . . 296 mg
Total Carbohydrate . . 3 g
   Dietary Fiber . . . . 1 g
   Sugars . . . . 1 g
Protein . . . . 23 g

4 4-oz lean mild fish filets, such as sole, rinsed and patted dry
1 oz sliced almonds (1/3 cup)
2 Tbsp reduced-fat margarine
2 Tbsp lemon juice
1 tsp Worcestershire sauce
1/2 tsp paprika
1/4 tsp salt
   Black pepper to taste

1. Heat oven to 375°F.
2. Coat a 9-inch by 13-inch baking pan with cooking spray. Arrange fish in pan. In a small bowl, combine almonds, margarine, lemon juice, Worcestershire, and paprika. Top filets with equal amounts of the almond mixture.
3. Bake 12–15 minutes or until fish is opaque in center. Sprinkle with salt and pepper and serve immediately.

Shrimp Pasta and Tomato Toss

It is important to assemble the tomato mixture first to allow the flavors to blend.

PREPARATION TIME
15 minutes

SERVES
4

SERVING SIZE
1/4 recipe

Exchanges

1 1/2 Starch

2 Very Lean Meat

1 Vegetable

Calories 214

   Calories from Fat. . . 30

Total Fat . . . . 3 g

   Saturated Fat . . . . . . 0 g

Cholesterol . . . . 142 mg

Sodium . . . . 400 mg

Total Carbohydrate . 26 g

   Dietary Fiber . . . . . . 2 g

   Sugars . . . . 3 g

Protein . . . . 20 g

1 1/2	cups diced plum tomatoes
16	kalamata olives, seeded and coarsely chopped
2	Tbsp chopped fresh basil or 2 tsp dried basil
1/8	tsp salt
4	oz uncooked spaghetti or fettucine, preferably spinach
1	lb raw unshelled shrimp or 13 oz (2 cups) raw, peeled, and deveined shrimp
1	medium lemon (about 1/4 cup juice)

1. In a small bowl, combine tomatoes, olives, basil, and salt. Toss to blend thoroughly and set aside. Peel and devein shrimp, if not already done.

2. Cook pasta in boiling water, omitting any salt or fat, for 7 minutes. Add shrimp and cook 3 minutes longer or until shrimp is opaque in center.

3. Drain pasta and shrimp in a colander and place on serving platter or in pasta bowl. Squeeze lemon over pasta and shrimp, top with tomato mixture, and toss gently, if desired.

Shrimp Steamer Bowl

This is a great dish to serve on a warm summer evening.

PREPARATION TIME
10 minutes

SERVES
4

SERVING SIZE
1/4 recipe

Exchanges

1 1/2 Starch

2 Very Lean Meat

1 Fat

Calories 219
   Calories from Fat. . . 64
Total Fat. . . . . 7 g
   Saturated Fat. . . . . . . 1 g
Cholesterol . . . . 142 mg
Sodium . . . . 494 mg
Total Carbohydrate . 23 g
   Dietary Fiber . . . . 3 g
   Sugars . . . . 2 g
Protein . . . . 18 g

1 lb raw unshelled shrimp or 13 oz (2 cups) raw, peeled, and deveined shrimp
4 2-oz new potatoes, cut in 8 wedges each
1 1/2 cups frozen corn kernels
1/4 cup reduced-fat margarine, melted
1 1/2 tsp seafood seasoning
1 medium lemon
   Black pepper to taste
2 Tbsp chopped fresh parsley

1. Peel and devein shrimp, if not already done. Place 2 cups water in a large saucepan, place collapsible steamer basket inside, and bring water to a boil.
2. Carefully place shrimp, potatoes, and corn in basket. Cover tightly and steam 10 minutes or until potatoes are just tender.
3. Meanwhile, in a small bowl, combine margarine and seafood seasoning and set aside.
4. When potatoes are cooked, carefully remove shrimp mixture from steamer basket and place on a shallow serving platter or pasta bowl. Add margarine mixture and toss gently, yet thoroughly, to coat completely. Squeeze fresh lemon over all and sprinkle with black pepper and parsley to serve.

Delicate Crab Frittata

Rinsing the canned crab gives a milder taste.

PREPARATION TIME
5 minutes

SERVES
4

SERVING SIZE
1/4 recipe

Exchanges

1/2 Carbohydrate

4 Very Lean Meat

1/2 Fat

Calories 188

   Calories from Fat . . . 47

Total Fat . . . . 5 g

   Saturated Fat . . . . 3 g

Cholesterol . . . . 70 mg

Sodium . . . . 734 mg

Total Carbohydrate . . 5 g

   Dietary Fiber . . . . 0 g

   Sugars . . . . 3 g

Protein . . . . 29 g

1 1/2 cups egg substitute (equal to 6 eggs)
1/3 cup evaporated fat-free milk
1/8 tsp cayenne pepper
1/8 tsp black pepper
2 6-oz cans white crab meat, lightly rinsed and drained in a fine mesh strainer
1/2 cup finely chopped green bell pepper
1/4 tsp salt
1/4 cup finely chopped green onion
3/4 cup shredded reduced-fat sharp cheddar cheese

1. In a small mixing bowl, combine egg substitute, evaporated milk, and peppers and whisk until smooth. Stir in crab and green pepper and set aside.
2. Heat a 12-inch nonstick skillet over medium heat. Add egg mixture, cover, and cook 10 minutes or until just slightly moist on top.
3. Remove from heat and sprinkle with salt, green onion, and cheese. Cover and let stand 3 minutes to allow cheese to melt and flavors to develop. Cut into 4 wedges and serve.

Speedy Sides

Does it seem like getting vegetables into your day is a chore? Eating enough vegetables is important, but you won't do it if it's not an easy and tasty experience. Take advantage of the prepared ingredients in your supermarket produce section: bagged lettuce mixes, baby carrots, prechopped items on the salad bar. Use bagged coleslaw mix in a quick stir-fry or steam baby carrots and toss them with a bit of butter. Introduce yourself to an incredibly vitamin-packed vegetable: bagged spinach. Place the spinach, all of it, in a hot skillet with a tiny amount of water and in less than a minute, your vegetable side is ready—simply season and serve!

To make vegetables more delicious, instead of boiling them, which leaches out the nutrients and waters down the flavor, try steaming or roasting them. Cut them in different ways—carrots diagonally or zucchini in long spears—to add interest to your plate. Serve green beans or tiny baby yellow squash or baby red potatoes whole.

Side dishes can dress up the simplest cuts of meat, or you can combine several sides for a meatless meal in minutes. Start with a few of the recipes in this chapter and see if your interest in vegetables awakens.

Spinach and Bacon

If you'd like to double this recipe, cook the spinach in two batches.

PREPARATION TIME
5 minutes

COOKING TIME
4 minutes

SERVES
4

SERVING SIZE
1/4 recipe

2 bacon slices, cut in very small pieces
1 pkg fresh spinach leaves
2 Tbsp water
1/8 tsp salt

1. Heat a 12-inch nonstick skillet over medium-high heat. Add bacon and cook until crisp. Remove bacon and blot on paper towels. Discard all but 2 tsp of the bacon grease.
2. Increase heat to high and add spinach, water, and salt to the 2 tsp bacon grease. Toss constantly until limp and tender, about 1 minute, using 2 utensils.
3. Remove from heat, crumble bacon on top, and serve.

Exchanges

1 Vegetable

1/2 Fat

Calories 53
  Calories from Fat. . . 34
Total Fat . . . . 4 g
  Saturated Fat . . . . 2 g
Cholesterol . . . . 5 mg
Sodium . . . . 171 mg
Total Carbohydrate . . 3 g
  Dietary Fiber . . . . 2 g
  Sugars . . . . 0 g
Protein . . . . 3 g

Sesame-Roasted Asparagus

You can sprinkle this asparagus with a little Parmesan cheese if you like.

PREPARATION TIME
5 minutes

SERVES
4

SERVING SIZE
1/4 recipe

1 lb asparagus spears, trimmed
2 tsp sesame seeds
1/8 tsp salt

1. Heat oven to 400°F.
2. Arrange asparagus on a nonstick baking sheet in a single layer. Lightly coat asparagus with cooking spray and sprinkle with sesame seeds and salt.
3. Bake 10–12 minutes until asparagus is just tender-crisp.

Exchanges

1 Vegetable

Calories 21
   Calories from Fat 8
Total Fat . . . . 1 g
   Saturated Fat . . . . 0 g
Cholesterol . . . . 0 mg
Sodium . . . . 82 mg
Total Carbohydrate . . 3 g
   Dietary Fiber . . . . 1 g
   Sugars . . . . 1 g
Protein . . . . 2 g

Dilled Whole Green Beans

Whole green beans are delicious with potatoes.

PREPARATION TIME
5 minutes

SERVES
4

SERVING SIZE
1/4 recipe

1 lb whole green beans, trimmed
1 Tbsp reduced-fat margarine
2 tsp Dijon mustard
1/2 tsp dried dill weed
1/8 tsp salt

1. Place 2 cups water in a large saucepan, place a collapsible steamer basket on bottom of pan, arrange beans evenly on basket, and cover tightly. Bring water to a boil and steam beans 6 minutes or until just tender-crisp.
2. In a small bowl, combine remaining ingredients.
3. Place cooked beans in a serving bowl and toss with the margarine mixture. Serve immediately.

Exchanges

1 Vegetable

1/2 Fat

Calories 48

Calories from Fat . . . 17

Total Fat . . . . 2 g

Saturated Fat . . . . 0 g

Cholesterol . . . . 0 mg

Sodium . . . . 157 mg

Total Carbohydrate . . 8 g

Dietary Fiber . . . . 3 g

Sugars . . . . 2 g

Protein . . . . 2 g

Honey-Roasted Carrot Wheels and Onions

Don't be tempted to substitute baby carrots in this recipe: they do not caramelize well.

PREPARATION TIME
10 minutes

SERVES
4

SERVING SIZE
1/4 recipe

12 oz carrots, peeled and cut into 1/4-inch slices
1 4-oz yellow onion, cut in 8 wedges
1 Tbsp honey
1 1/2 tsp vegetable oil
1/8 tsp salt

1. Heat oven to 450°F.
2. Place carrots and onions on a nonstick baking sheet and drizzle honey and oil evenly over all. Using 2 spoons, toss gently to coat carrots, then arrange in a single layer.
3. Bake 10 minutes, then stir and bake 5 minutes longer or until carrots are tender-crisp and richly browned. Sprinkle with salt to serve.

Exchanges

1 Carbohydrate

Calories 74
  Calories from Fat . . . 17
Total Fat . . . . 2 g
  Saturated Fat . . . . 0 g
Cholesterol . . . . 0 mg
Sodium . . . . 173 mg
Total Carbohydrate . 14 g
  Dietary Fiber . . . . 3 g
  Sugars . . . . 10 g
Protein . . . . 1 g

Broiled Blue Cheese Romas

You'll like the flavor of Roma tomatoes in this recipe, but it will work just as well with regular tomatoes.

PREPARATION TIME
5 minutes

SERVES
4

SERVING SIZE
1/4 recipe

Exchanges

1 Vegetable

1/2 Fat

Calories 42

   Calories from Fat. . . 20

Total Fat . . . . 2 g

   Saturated Fat . . . . . . 1 g

Cholesterol . . . . 5 mg

Sodium . . . . 258 mg

Total Carbohydrate . . 4 g

   Dietary Fiber . . . . 1 g

   Sugars . . . . 3 g

Protein . . . . 2 g

  4 Roma or plum tomatoes, halved lengthwise
  2 Tbsp fat-free Italian salad dressing
1/2 tsp dried basil
1/8 tsp salt
1/8 tsp pepper
  1 oz blue cheese, crumbled

1. Heat broiler.
2. Arrange tomatoes on a nonstick baking sheet, cut side up. Drizzle dressing evenly over tomatoes, about 3/4 tsp per tomato half, then sprinkle with basil.
3. Broil 2–3 inches away from heat source for 1 minute. Remove tomatoes from broiler and top with salt, pepper, and cheese.
4. Return to broiler, turn off heat, and let stand in oven 3 minutes or until cheese just begins to turn light golden.

Cheddar'd Yellow Squash

. Try this recipe with zucchini, too.

PREPARATION TIME
5 minutes

SERVES
4

SERVING SIZE
1/4 recipe

4   4-oz yellow squash, cut in half lengthwise
1/4   cup finely chopped green onion
1/8   tsp salt
Black pepper to taste
1/2   cup shredded reduced-fat sharp cheddar cheese

1. Heat oven to 400°F.
2. Coat a nonstick baking sheet with cooking spray and arrange squash cut side up on baking sheet.
3. Lightly coat squash with cooking spray and top each half with 1 1/2 tsp onion. Sprinkle salt and pepper evenly over all, top with cheese, and bake 20 minutes or until cheese melts.

Exchanges

1 Vegetable

1 Fat

Calories 64
   Calories from Fat . . . 29
Total Fat . . . . 3 g
   Saturated Fat . . . . . . 2 g
Cholesterol . . . . 10 mg
Sodium . . . . 198 mg
Total Carbohydrate . . 5 g
   Dietary Fiber . . . . 2 g
   Sugars . . . . 3 g
Protein . . . . 5 g

Broccoli with Spicy Cheese Sauce

You can spice up this cheese sauce as much as you like!

PREPARATION TIME
5 minutes

SERVES
4

SERVING SIZE
1 cup

4	cups broccoli florets
4	slices reduced-fat American cheese
2	tsp fat-free milk
1/2	tsp Worcestershire sauce
1/8–1/4	tsp cayenne pepper

1. Place 2 cups water in a large saucepan, place a collapsible steamer basket on bottom of pan, arrange florets evenly on basket, and cover tightly. Bring water to a boil and steam broccoli 5–6 minutes or until just tender-crisp.
2. When broccoli has cooked, place cheese slices in a microwaveable bowl, cover with plastic wrap, and microwave on HIGH setting 45 seconds or until cheese has melted. Stir in remaining ingredients.
3. Arrange broccoli on a serving platter, drizzle sauce over broccoli, and serve immediately.

Exchanges

1 Lean Meat

1 Vegetable

Calories 79
   Calories from Fat. . . 29
Total Fat. . . . . 3 g
   Saturated Fat. . . . . . . 2 g
Cholesterol . . . . 10 mg
Sodium . . . . 326 mg
Total Carbohydrate . . 7 g
   Dietary Fiber . . . . 3 g
   Sugars . . . . 3 g
Protein . . . . 7 g

Free Veggie Stir-Fry

Use different veggies to change the flavor of this quick stir-fry—try mushrooms, zucchini, and carrots next time.

PREPARATION TIME
5 minutes

SERVES
4

SERVING SIZE
1/4 recipe

1	6-oz yellow squash, trimmed and cut into eighths lengthwise
1/2	medium green bell pepper, cut in thin strips
4	oz yellow onion, cut in 1/2-inch wedges, layers separated
1/8–1/4	tsp salt

1. Heat a 12-inch nonstick skillet over medium-high heat. Coat skillet with nonstick cooking spray. Add vegetables and cook 3 minutes, stirring constantly.
2. Add salt and cook 1 minute longer or until just tender-crisp.
3. Remove from heat and let stand 1 minute before serving.

Exchanges

1 Vegetable

Calories 22
   Calories from Fat. . . . 2
Total Fat. . . . . 0 g
   Saturated Fat. . . . . . . 0 g
Cholesterol . . . . 0 mg
Sodium . . . . 77 mg
Total Carbohydrate . . 5 g
   Dietary Fiber . . . . 1 g
   Sugars. . . . . 3 g
Protein . . . . 1 g

Sweet Potatoes with Orange Marmalade

Cinnamon adds great flavor and color to this yummy topping.

2 8-oz sweet potatoes, pierced several times
1 1/2 Tbsp reduced-fat margarine
1 1/2 Tbsp orange marmalade
1/2 tsp ground cinnamon

1. Place potatoes in microwave and cook on HIGH setting for 6 minutes or until tender when pierced with a fork.
2. Meanwhile, in a small mixing bowl, combine remaining ingredients and set aside.
3. When potatoes are done, split in half lengthwise, fluff potatoes with a fork, and spoon equal amounts (about 2 tsp each) of the marmalade mixture on top of each potato half.

Exchanges

1 1/2 Starch

Calories 124
   Calories from Fat . . . 21
Total Fat . . . . 2 g
   Saturated Fat . . . . 0 g
Cholesterol . . . . 0 mg
Sodium . . . . 39 mg
Total Carbohydrate . 25 g
   Dietary Fiber . . . . 3 g
   Sugars . . . . 13 g
Protein . . . . 2 g

Greek Potato Wedges

It's better to add the parsley after the potatoes have stood for 3 minutes; it will give a more pronounced fresh herb flavor.

PREPARATION TIME
5 minutes

SERVES
4

SERVING SIZE
1/4 recipe

1 lb new red potatoes (about 2 oz each), cut into 1/2-inch wedges
2 Tbsp extra virgin olive oil
1/2 tsp lemon pepper seasoning
1/2 tsp dried oregano
1/8 tsp salt
2 Tbsp chopped fresh parsley

1. Place 2 cups water in a large saucepan, place a collapsible steamer basket on bottom of pan, arrange potato wedges evenly on basket, and cover tightly. Bring water to a boil and steam potatoes 8 minutes or until just tender.
2. Place potatoes in a serving bowl and toss gently with oil, lemon pepper seasoning, oregano, and salt. Cover and let stand 3 minutes to absorb flavors.
3. Sprinkle with parsley and serve.

Exchanges

1 1/2 Starch

1 Fat

Calories 146
    Calories from Fat . . . 55
Total Fat . . . . 6 g
    Saturated Fat . . . . 1 g
Cholesterol . . . . 0 mg
Sodium . . . . 129 mg
Total Carbohydrate . 21 g
    Dietary Fiber . . . . 2 g
    Sugars . . . . 2 g
Protein . . . . 3 g

Rough Potato Mash

The texture of these potatoes is wonderfully lumpy.

PREPARATION TIME
5 minutes

SERVES
5

SERVING SIZE
1/2 cup

1 lb unpeeled Russet potatoes, diced
1/2 cup evaporated fat-free milk
2 Tbsp reduced-fat margarine
1/4 cup light sour cream
1/8 tsp garlic powder
1/4 tsp salt
1/8 tsp black pepper

1. Place 2 cups water in a large saucepan, place a collapsible steamer basket on bottom of pan, arrange potatoes evenly on basket, and cover tightly. Bring water to a boil and steam potatoes 8 minutes or until just tender.

2. Place potatoes in a serving bowl and, using a whisk, mash potatoes. Add remaining ingredients and whisk until well blended. The texture will be a bit lumpy.

Exchanges

1 Starch
1/2 Fat

Calories 115
   Calories from Fat . . . 31
Total Fat . . . . 3 g
   Saturated Fat . . . . . . 1 g
Cholesterol . . . . 4 mg
Sodium . . . . 174 mg
Total Carbohydrate . 18 g
   Dietary Fiber . . . . . . 2 g
   Sugars . . . . 3 g
Protein . . . . 4 g

Pasta with Basil and Parmesan

I like to use vermicelli in this recipe.

PREPARATION TIME
5 minutes

SERVES
4

SERVING SIZE
1/2 cup

4 oz uncooked pasta, any shape
1 Tbsp lemon juice
1 Tbsp finely chopped fresh parsley
2 tsp extra virgin olive oil
1 tsp dried basil
1/4 tsp salt
2 Tbsp grated Parmesan cheese

1. Cook pasta according to package directions, omitting any salt or fat.
2. Meanwhile, in a small bowl, combine remaining ingredients except Parmesan.
3. Place pasta in serving bowl and toss with lemon mixture. Sprinkle with Parmesan and serve immediately.

Exchanges

1 1/2 Starch

1/2 Fat

Calories 140
    Calories from Fat . . . 33
Total Fat . . . . 4 g
    Saturated Fat . . . . 1 g
Cholesterol . . . . 4 mg
Sodium . . . . 210 mg
Total Carbohydrate . 22 g
    Dietary Fiber . . . . 1 g
    Sugars . . . . 1 g
Protein . . . . 5 g

Cheesy Risotto with Onions

Try this great side dish with pork tenderloin.

PREPARATION TIME
5 minutes

SERVES
6

SERVING SIZE
1/2 cup

1 3/4 cups water
  3/4 cup uncooked brown or white rice
    2 cups chopped yellow onion
    3 oz shredded reduced-fat sharp
      cheddar cheese (3/4 cup)
  1/4 tsp garlic powder
  1/8 tsp cayenne pepper
  3/4 tsp salt
  1/8 tsp black pepper

1. Boil water in a medium saucepan and stir in rice and onion. Cover and simmer 35 minutes for brown rice, 20 minutes for white rice, or until rice is tender, but with a small amount of liquid remaining.
2. Remove from heat and stir in remaining ingredients until well blended. Cover and let stand 2–3 minutes to develop flavors.

Exchanges

1 1/2 Starch

Calories 146
  Calories from Fat . . . 34
Total Fat . . . . 4 g
  Saturated Fat . . . . 2 g
Cholesterol . . . . 10 mg
Sodium . . . . 414 mg
Total Carbohydrate . 23 g
  Dietary Fiber . . . . 2 g
  Sugars . . . . 4 g
Protein . . . . 6 g

Easy-Does-It Desserts

If you haven't heard, desserts are no longer off limits for people with diabetes! Just account for the dessert carbohydrate in your daily total, and, of course, indulge with moderation. Remember that you can freeze most dessert leftovers to use another day—a great way to keep temptation at bay.

The easy sweets in this chapter are great-tasting, but take only a few minutes to make. They provide that wonderful homemade flavor, but with much less fat, calories, and time involved.

For example, to whip up a quick berry pie, simply quick-cook your favorite fruit and spices in a skillet while the piecrust bakes ... slide the crust on top of the fruit in the skillet and you're done ... in no time!

Angel Cake with Raspberry Cream and Nectarines

A serrated knife works best to cut angel food cake slices.

PREPARATION TIME
5 minutes

SERVES
4

SERVING SIZE
1/4 recipe

3/4 cup fat-free whipped topping
3 Tbsp all-fruit seedless raspberry spread
1/4 tsp almond extract
4 oz angel food cake (about 1/4 of a standard angel food cake), cut in 4 slices
2 cups sliced nectarines or peaches

1. In a small mixing bowl, mix together whipped topping with fruit spread and extract.
2. Spoon equal amounts (about 2 Tbsp) over each slice of cake and top with 1/2 cup nectarine slices per serving.

Exchanges

2 1/2 Carbohydrate

Calories 162
   Calories from Fat. 3
Total Fat. . . . . 0 g
   Saturated Fat. . . . . . . 0 g
Cholesterol . . . . 0 mg
Sodium . . . . 62 mg
Total Carbohydrate . 37 g
   Dietary Fiber . . . . 2 g
   Sugars . . . . 23 g
Protein . . . . 3 g

Warm Shortcakes with Orange'd Strawberries

This is the perfect summer dessert.

PREPARATION TIME
15 minutes

SERVES
8

SERVING SIZE
1 shortcake

Exchanges

2 1/2 Carbohydrate

1/2 Fat

Calories 203

   Calories from Fat. . . 52

Total Fat. . . . . 6 g

   Saturated Fat. . . . . . . 1 g

Cholesterol . . . . 1 mg

Sodium . . . . 482 mg

Total Carbohydrate . 36 g

   Dietary Fiber . . . . 3 g

   Sugars. . . . . 14 g

Protein . . . . 5 g

4 cups sliced strawberries
3 Tbsp sugar, divided
1/2 tsp orange zest
   Juice of medium orange
2 1/4 cups reduced-fat biscuit baking mix
1 cup fat-free plain yogurt
1/4 cup reduced-fat margarine
1 cup fat-free whipped topping (optional)

1. Heat oven to 425°F.
2. In a gallon zippered plastic bag, combine strawberries, 1 Tbsp sugar, orange zest, and orange juice. Seal tightly, releasing any excess air, and press gently to mash some of the strawberries in order to thicken the mixture slightly. Set aside.
3. In a medium mixing bowl, combine baking mix, yogurt, margarine, and the remaining sugar. Stir until well blended.
4. Spoon the batter onto a nonstick baking sheet in 8 mounds and bake 10–12 minutes or until lightly golden.
5. Place shortcakes in individual bowls, spoon 1/2 cup strawberries over each shortcake, and top each with 2 Tbsp whipped topping, if desired.

Pineapple Gingerbread Squares

Try this moist, delicious cake for the holidays—the smell of baking gingerbread will warm your spirits! It tastes even better the next day.

PREPARATION TIME
5 minutes

SERVES
24

SERVING SIZE
1 square

1 14.5-oz box gingerbread cake and cookie mix
2 8-oz cans crushed pineapple in its own juice
2 4-oz jars baby food pureed carrots
1/2 cup quick-cooking oats
1 large egg

1. Heat oven to 350°F.
2. Add all ingredients to a 9-inch by 13-inch nonstick baking pan and stir until well blended. Bake 30 minutes or until wooden toothpick inserted in center comes out clean.
3. Place on cooling rack and allow to cool completely before cutting.

Exchanges

1 Carbohydrate

1/2 Fat

Calories 96

Calories from Fat . . . 21

Total Fat . . . . 2 g

Saturated Fat . . . . 1 g

Cholesterol . . . . 9 mg

Sodium . . . . 124 mg

Total Carbohydrate . 17 g

Dietary Fiber . . . . 1 g

Sugars . . . . 9 g

Protein . . . . 1 g

Caramel Walnut Brownies

The oats make these brownies thick and chewy.

PREPARATION TIME
5 minutes

SERVES
24

SERVING SIZE
1 brownie

1 20.5-oz pkg reduced-fat brownie mix
1 cup quick-cooking oats
1 cup water
2 oz walnut or pecan pieces
 (about 1/2 cup)
2 Tbsp fat-free caramel or butterscotch
 ice cream topping

1. Heat oven to 350°F.
2. In a mixing bowl, combine brownie mix, oats, and
 water and blend well. Spoon batter into a 9-inch by
 13-inch nonstick baking pan, top with walnuts,
 and bake 25 minutes or until wooden toothpick
 inserted in center comes out almost clean.
3. Place on wire rack and let cool completely.
4. Drizzle caramel on top of brownies and cut.

Exchanges

1 1/2 Carbohydrate

1/2 Fat

Calories 133
   Calories from Fat. . . 23
Total Fat . . . . 3 g
   Saturated Fat. . . . . . . 0 g
Cholesterol . . . . 0 mg
Sodium . . . . 92 mg
Total Carbohydrate . 26 g
   Dietary Fiber . . . . 0 g
   Sugars . . . . 17 g
Protein . . . . 2 g

Patty Cake Cookies

Use alternate baking sheets to allow each sheet to cool down completely between batches.

PREPARATION TIME
15 minutes

SERVES
48

SERVING SIZE
1 cookie

Exchanges

1/2 Carbohydrate

Calories 54
   Calories from Fat . . . 13
Total Fat . . . . 1 g
   Saturated Fat . . . . 0 g
Cholesterol . . . . 0 mg
Sodium . . . . 76 mg
Total Carbohydrate . 10 g
   Dietary Fiber . . . . 0 g
   Sugars . . . . 6 g
Protein . . . . 1 g

1 18.25-oz box white cake mix
1/4 cup egg substitute
1 6-oz jar baby food pureed pears
2 Tbsp vegetable oil
1 Tbsp lemon zest
3 Tbsp all-fruit raspberry or apricot spread

1. Heat oven to 375°F.
2. In a large mixing bowl, combine all ingredients except fruit spread and stir until well blended, using a rubber spatula to break up lumps.
3. Spoon batter by level tablespoons about 2 inches apart onto a nonstick baking sheet and bake 7–10 minutes or until edges are just slightly golden. Remove from oven and let stand on baking sheet 2 full minutes before removing. Cool completely. Repeat until all batter is used.
4. When cookies are completely cooled, place fruit spread in a small bowl. Using a fork, whisk until smooth and pliable. Top each cookie with 1/4 tsp spread.

Rustic Apple Crisp

The flavors blend beautifully in this easy apple crisp.

PREPARATION TIME
10 minutes

SERVES
8

SERVING SIZE
1/8 recipe

2 oz pecan chips (smaller than pieces)
1 lb Granny Smith apples, unpeeled (about 5 cups sliced)
2 Tbsp water
1/2 tsp ground cinnamon
1/4 cup fat-free caramel ice cream topping, divided
2 cups low-fat granola cereal

1. Heat a 12-inch nonstick skillet over medium-high heat. Add pecans and cook 4 minutes or until just beginning to turn golden and fragrant, stirring frequently. Remove from skillet and set aside on separate plate.
2. Cut apples in half, core, and cut in 1/2-inch wedges. Return skillet to heat. Add apples and water and cook, uncovered, 4 minutes or until just tender-crisp, stirring frequently.
3. Remove skillet from heat and sprinkle cinnamon over apples. Drizzle 1 Tbsp caramel topping over apples and stir gently. Top with granola, cover, and let stand 1 minute to absorb flavors.
4. Place remaining caramel topping in a microwaveable bowl and microwave on HIGH setting for 15 seconds. Drizzle over granola and top with nuts to serve.

Exchanges

2 1/2 Carbohydrate

1 Fat

Calories 206
   Calories from Fat . . . 55
Total Fat . . . . 6 g
   Saturated Fat . . . . 0 g
Cholesterol . . . . 0 mg
Sodium . . . . 88 mg
Total Carbohydrate . 37 g
   Dietary Fiber . . . . 4 g
   Sugars . . . . 19 g
Protein . . . . 3 g

Double Berry Pie

Remove any leftovers from the skillet and place in a pie pan. Cover with plastic wrap and store at room temperature up to 48 hours. Leftovers have a rustic cobbler look.

PREPARATION TIME
10 minutes

SERVES
10

SERVING SIZE
1 piece

Exchanges

2 Carbohydrate

1 Fat

Calories	177
Calories from Fat . . .	52
Total Fat	6 g
Saturated Fat	2 g
Cholesterol	4 mg
Sodium	83 mg
Total Carbohydrate .	31 g
Dietary Fiber	1 g
Sugars	16 g
Protein	1 g

1 refrigerated pie crust dough
1/2 cup plus 1 Tbsp sugar
1/2 tsp ground cinnamon, divided
1 16-oz can tart pitted cherries with liquid or 12-oz bag frozen raspberries
2 cups frozen blueberries
3 Tbsp cornstarch
1/2 tsp vanilla or 1/4 tsp almond extract

1. Heat oven to 450°F.
2. Follow package directions for bringing pie crust to room temperature in the microwave.
3. Place pie crust on a nonstick baking sheet. Using a fork, pierce the pie crust in several places to prevent puffing and bake 7–8 minutes or until lightly golden.
4. In a small bowl, combine 1/4 tsp cinnamon with 1 Tbsp sugar and set aside.
5. Meanwhile, place cherries and liquid, blueberries, 1/2 cup sugar, cornstarch, and 1/4 tsp cinnamon in a 12-inch nonstick skillet over high heat. Gently stir with a rubber spatula until cornstarch completely dissolves. Bring to a boil, stirring frequently. Continue to boil 1–2 minutes or until thickened, scraping bottom and sides of skillet. Remove from heat and stir in extract.
6. Remove pie crust, coat with cooking spray, and sprinkle with cinnamon sugar. Place crust on top of fruit in skillet to serve.

Devil's Food Ice Cream Pie

Best to add chocolate syrup after freezing pie—otherwise, the chocolate flavor is not as pronounced.

PREPARATION TIME
15 minutes

SERVES
10

SERVING SIZE
1 piece

Exchanges

2 Carbohydrate

1 Fat

Calories 191

   Calories from Fat. . . 55

Total Fat . . . . 6 g

   Saturated Fat . . . . 3 g

Cholesterol . . . . 20 mg

Sodium . . . . 112 mg

Total Carbohydrate . 32 g

   Dietary Fiber . . . . 1 g

   Sugars . . . . 18 g

Protein . . . . 5 g

1 6 3/4-oz box devil's food cookie cakes (12 cookies)
1/4 cup reduced-fat peanut butter
1/4 cup water
1 cup sliced bananas
4 cups no-sugar-added light vanilla ice cream
2 Tbsp chocolate syrup

1. Break cookies into 1/2-inch pieces. (You may want to coat your fingertips with cooking spray to reduce the stickiness when handling cookies.) Place cookie pieces in bottom of a 9-inch deep dish pie pan.
2. Place peanut butter and water in a medium microwaveable bowl, cover with plastic wrap, and cook on HIGH setting for 20 seconds. Remove from microwave, whisk until completely smooth, and drizzle evenly over cookies.
3. Top with banana slices and carefully spoon ice cream evenly over all. Cover with plastic wrap and place in freezer until firm, about 8 hours.
4. At time of serving, drizzle chocolate syrup over all.

Frozen Peach Cream

Let the solidly frozen dessert stand at room temperature for 15 minutes before serving.

PREPARATION TIME
5 minutes

SERVES
8

SERVING SIZE
1/2 cup

2 cups no-sugar-added light vanilla ice cream
1 lb bag frozen peaches, partially thawed
1/2 cup white grape peach juice (100% juice)
1/4 cup all-fruit seedless raspberry spread

1. Place all ingredients in a food processor and process until smooth. If using a blender, work in two batches.
2. Place in a plastic container and freeze 30 minutes for a semi-soft texture or 2 hours for a firmer consistency.

Exchanges
1 Carbohydrate
1/2 Fat

Calories 94
   Calories from Fat . . . 21
Total Fat . . . . 2 g
   Saturated Fat . . . . 1 g
Cholesterol . . . . 13 mg
Sodium . . . . 29 mg
Total Carbohydrate . 18 g
   Dietary Fiber . . . . 1 g
   Sugars . . . . 13 g
Protein . . . . 2 g

Cranberry Wine Ice

This stores well in the freezer for one month. Because of the alcohol, the mixture will not freeze solid.

PREPARATION TIME
3 minutes

SERVES
12

SERVING SIZE
1/2 cup

2 cups cranberry-raspberry juice (100% juice)
1 cup merlot or any dry red wine
1/2 cup frozen purple grape juice concentrate

1. Place all ingredients in a 2-qt plastic container with lid and freeze overnight or at least 8 hours until firm.
2. Lightly stir with a fork before serving.

Exchanges

1 Carbohydrate

Calories 62
　Calories from Fat 1
Total Fat . . . . 0 g
　Saturated Fat . . . . 0 g
Cholesterol . . . . 0 mg
Sodium . . . . 9 mg
Total Carbohydrate . 12 g
　Dietary Fiber . . . . 0 g
　Sugars . . . . 12 g
Protein . . . . 0 g

Mocha-Drizzled Flan

To boil water in the microwave, place 2 cups water in a microwaveable container and microwave on HIGH setting for 3 minutes or until the water comes to a boil.

PREPARATION TIME
10 minutes

SERVES
6

SERVING SIZE
1/6 recipe

Exchanges

1 1/2 Carbohydrate

1 Lean Meat

Calories 154
   Calories from Fat. . . 24
Total Fat . . . . 3 g
   Saturated Fat. . . . . . 1 g
Cholesterol . . . . 107 mg
Sodium . . . . 143 mg
Total Carbohydrate . 23 g
   Dietary Fiber . . . . 0 g
   Sugars . . . . 20 g
Protein . . . . 10 g

1 1/2 cups evaporated fat-free milk
3 large eggs
3 egg whites
1/3 cup sugar
1 tsp vanilla/butter/nut-flavored extract, divided
2 cups boiling water
1/4 tsp instant coffee granules
1 Tbsp water
2 Tbsp chocolate syrup

1. Heat oven to 325°F.
2. In a medium bowl, combine milk, eggs, egg whites, sugar, and 1/2 tsp extract and whisk together until well blended.
3. Coat 6 6-oz pyrex ramekins with cooking spray and set in a 9-inch by 13-inch baking pan. Pour equal amounts of the egg mixture in each of the six ramekins and place pan on center rack of oven. Pour the boiling water in pan around ramekins. Bake 40 minutes or until knife inserted in center comes out clean.
4. While flan is baking, in a small bowl combine coffee and water and stir until granules have dissolved. Add chocolate syrup and remaining 1/2 tsp extract and stir until well blended.
5. Remove cooked flans from oven and place on wire racks to cool slightly. Insert knife and slide around outer edges to release custard. Place dessert plate over each ramekin and invert. Spoon equal amounts of the sauce around outer edges of each flan, about 1 1/2 tsp per serving.

Easy Summer Strawberries

Serve these in frozen wine goblets when you're entertaining.

PREPARATION TIME
3 minutes

SERVES
6

SERVING SIZE
1/6 recipe

4 cups strawberries or combination of strawberries, blueberries and raspberries, rinsed and patted dry

1/4 cup frozen purple grape juice concentrate

1/2 tsp vanilla or almond extract

In a medium mixing bowl, combine all ingredients and toss gently. Serve immediately.

Exchanges

1 Fruit

Calories 57
   Calories from Fat 4
Total Fat . . . . 0 g
   Saturated Fat . . . . 0 g
Cholesterol . . . . 0 mg
Sodium . . . . 5 mg
Total Carbohydrate . 14 g
   Dietary Fiber . . . . 2 g
   Sugars . . . . 11 g
Protein . . . . 1 g

Honey-Glazed Almond Pears

Watch out—if you wait longer than 30 minutes to serve this dessert, the almonds will soften and the flavors will begin to fade!

PREPARATION TIME
5 minutes

SERVES
4

SERVING SIZE
1/4 recipe

Exchanges

1 1/2 Carbohydrate

1 Fat

Calories 127

   Calories from Fat . . . 34

Total Fat . . . . 4 g

   Saturated Fat . . . . 0 g

Cholesterol . . . . 0 mg

Sodium . . . . 20 mg

Total Carbohydrate . 25 g

   Dietary Fiber . . . . 3 g

   Sugars . . . . 21 g

Protein . . . . 1 g

1/2 oz sliced almonds (scant 3 Tbsp)
2 Tbsp honey
2 8-oz pears, cut in half lengthwise and cored
1 Tbsp reduced-fat margarine
1/2 tsp vanilla extract

1. Heat a 12-inch nonstick skillet over medium-high heat. Add almonds and cook 4 minutes or until lightly browned, stirring frequently. Remove almonds from skillet.

2. Reduce heat to medium and add honey. Arrange pear halves, cut side down, on top of honey and cook 6 minutes or until pears are just tender. Remove skillet from heat and place pears, cut side up, on serving platter.

3. Stir margarine and vanilla into the pan drippings until well blended. Stir in almonds and spoon equal amounts over each pear half. Let cool to room temperature to allow flavors to blend before serving, about 30 minutes.

Index

Alphabetical List of Recipes

Subject Index

About the American Diabetes Association

The American Diabetes Association is the nation's leading voluntary health organization supporting diabetes research, information, and advocacy. Its mission is to prevent and cure diabetes and to improve the lives of all people affected by diabetes. The American Diabetes Association is the leading publisher of comprehensive diabetes information. Its huge library of practical and authoritative books for people with diabetes covers every aspect of self-care—cooking and nutrition, fitness, weight control, medications, complications, emotional issues, and general self-care.

To order American Diabetes Association books: Call 1-800-232-6733. http://store.diabetes.org [Note: there is no need to use **www** when typing this particular Web address]

To join the American Diabetes Association: Call 1-800-806-7801. www.diabetes.org/membership

For more information about diabetes or ADA programs and services: Call 1-800-342-2383. E-mail: Customerservice@diabetes.org

To locate an ADA/NCQA Recognized Provider of quality diabetes care in your area: Call 1-703-549-1500 ext. 2202. www.diabetes.org/recognition/Physicians/ListAll.asp

To find an ADA Recognized Education Program in your area: Call 1-888-232-0822. www.diabetes.org/recognition/education.asp

To join the fight to increase funding for diabetes research, end discrimination, and improve insurance coverage: Call 1-800-342-2383. www.diabetes.org/advocacy

To find out how you can get involved with the programs in your community: Call 1-800-342-2383. See below for program Web addresses.

- *American Diabetes Month:* Educational activities aimed at those diagnosed with diabetes—month of November. www.diabetes.org/ADM

- *American Diabetes Alert:* Annual public awareness campaign to find the undiagnosed— held the fourth Tuesday in March. www.diabetes.org/alert

- *The Diabetes Assistance & Resources Program (DAR):* diabetes awareness program targeted to the Latino community. www.diabetes.org/DAR

- *African American Program:* diabetes awareness program targeted to the African American community. www.diabetes.org/africanamerican

- *Awakening the Spirit: Pathways to Diabetes Prevention & Control:* diabetes awareness program targeted to the Native American community. www.diabetes.org/awakening

To find out about an important research project regarding type 2 diabetes: www.diabetes.org/ada/research.asp

To obtain information on making a planned gift or charitable bequest: Call 1-888-700-7029. www.diabetes.org/ada/plan.asp

To make a donation or memorial contribution: Call 1-800-342-2383. www.diabetes.org/ada/cont.asp